Run With It

A True Story of Parkinson's, Marathons, the Pandemic, and Love

Joe Drake

Some commercially-available products are mentioned herein. Such mentions
are made without the knowledge of the products' manufacturers and the
author has received no compensation in return.

On April 1, 2022, well after the events described herein and before
publication of this book, the author was chosen by the HOKA company to
serve as a field ambassador for their product line (aka HOKA Flyer).

The author is not a physician. Any readers inspired to emulate any
of his athletic pursuits are strongly advised to consult with
their medical care teams beforehand.

Book cover artwork was created by Patricia Snyder.

To my wife, Lynn, who has brought me
a life filled with love and adventure.

And to my son, Aidan, and my daughter, Kinsey,
who have always made fatherhood a joy for me.

All profits from the sale of this book
earned by the author will be donated
to The Michael J. Fox Foundation
for Parkinson's Research.

Contents

Preface

For decades now, I've had in my mind the idea of running a marathon. It's a thought that I suppose many runners find difficult to dismiss. The marathon has such allure: the challenge, the demonstration of fitness and courage, the bright shiny medal, the hard-earned postrace beer, and so on. Until recently, though, this idea never reached the level of a goal for me. Had it done so, I believe that I would've achieved it long ago. Then, it was only just an idea albeit a tenacious one.

I've felt similarly about writing a book. At times I even started in on one. But the words never flowed freely enough to make the effort worthwhile. Character development, a compelling plot, poignant insights into human nature—all these elements of a good story eluded me. My skills, it seemed, were best suited to the genre of well-crafted emails.

It took a diagnosis of Parkinson's disease to unite these disparate inclinations of mine. Life can take such magnificent and mysterious turns.

Here's another puzzle. Why is it, I ask myself, that it's taken me six decades, including an engineering career immersed in science, data, and documentation, before realizing that fiction is not my strength? Writers should write of what they know. Yet, it's only been in the past year that I've heard that voice in my head say, "You are living the story now. Write it down!"

I've written it down. A perfect storm of Parkinson's, vigorous exercise as an effective therapy for the disease, and the COVID-19 pandemic blew me off my quiet course into an adventure so rich and so fun that I feel it's worth sharing. Along the way I stumbled onto a strategy for dealing with a pernicious disease that as yet has no cure. I hope this book resonates with those newly diagnosed with Parkinson's disease and with others who have lived with the disease for years. There's hope for those who are willing to put in some effort.

Runners may also find this book engaging. In it I describe my transformation into a marathoner, and I detail my effort to run the World Marathon Majors amidst a world eager to emerge from a global catastrophe. Don't mistake it for a complete guide to distance running, however, as there are better resources elsewhere and I cite some of them here for those who aren't already experts. To be sure, I cringe somewhat at the thought of highly experienced runners getting a hearty belly laugh at some of my mistakes. That's not to say I don't want them to read this book. On the contrary. I would be honored if they did. I write here about how running is excellent therapy but, hey, so is laughter.

If this book were only about Parkinson's and running, however, it might never have been written. Friends, family, and other acquaintances have convinced me that there's a universal element of the inspirational also at play in my story.

I'm one of those people who gets emotional when witnessing acts of courage and determination. Demonstrations of the human spirit can be profoundly beautiful. The world of sport is full of such acts.

The following come to mind:

Kerri Strug at the 1996 Olympics, her ankle badly sprained on her first vault, sticks an excruciatingly painful landing on her second attempt to clinch the gold medal for her team.

Wayne Rooney, the legendary English footballer well past his prime and now playing for the American Major League Soccer club DC United, sprints down three-quarters of the pitch to tackle an opponent on a breakaway, gets up, brings the ball back up the field himself, and sends a beautiful cross to his teammate whose header wins the game in stoppage time.

Alex Smith undergoes 17 surgeries on his horrifically mangled right leg, wills himself through an improbable rehabilitation, and comes back to quarterback his Washington Football Team to the division title.

I get choked up just reading through these last paragraphs. I feel the same way reading certain passages in this book. I'm not referring to my own exploits— that would be immodest. I'm referring to the actions of so many heroes I met during this journey.

All of us have the ability to inspire and to be inspired.

Enjoy.

Joe Drake
Seattle, Washington
July 2022

1

Halfway There

I was in Chicago's Jackson Street transit station entering the pivotal leg of my adventure—the journey back to Boston. Timing was critical but, frustrated, I couldn't stop the minutes from slipping away. That power belonged to the Chicago Transit Authority and its fickle Blue Line 'L' train that refused to show.

I had misjudged some key parameters. My wave's start time for the Chicago Marathon was 7:30 am and I allowed for five hours to run the race. That was nearly half an hour longer than I needed in London the week before. Should have been plenty of time. But I didn't account for the 15 minutes it would take to reach the starting line once my wave was sent off. Also, the heat and humidity were even worse than during my farcical performance in the Berlin race two weeks prior. The uncooperative weather forced me to walk more of the Chicago route than I intended and, hence, five hours was not enough time after all.

All told the race ate up 30 minutes of the buffer time I gave myself for returning to O'Hare Airport. The wait at Jackson consumed another 30. Missing that plane would almost certainly doom my entry into the Boston Marathon the next day. Dang it! What a mess. I should've booked a later flight to give myself more time in Chicago. I gambled, though, thinking it imperative to get to Boston as early as possible to prepare for that race.

I ran through the timing again as the train finally pulled into Jackson. My flight on United was to depart at 3:40 pm and it was closing in on 2 o'clock. Transit to the airport normally takes an hour so that left me 40 minutes to get to the gate. Is that enough time? What else could go wrong?

The day before on my way into downtown there was a work slowdown at Montrose (or was it Rosemont?) that held the train up for at least five minutes. Likely to happen on the return trip too, so the 40 minutes drops down to 35 minutes at best. Plus, the Chicago Marathon wiped me out—just walking to the station nearly did me in. I felt like shit, I couldn't walk very fast, and I wasn't thinking clearly. I figured I'd be wasting 10 or so foggy minutes stumbling around O'Hare until I got the lay of the land. Then I would need, maybe, 15 minutes to get through security. At what point would they stop allowing passengers to board? How much time do I have left to reach the gate? Damn! If I got to the gate on time, it would be very close.

With my leg cramps and nausea and suitcase and a station full of other O'Hare-destined marathoners, it was a struggle to board the train and find a seat. But I did get one, fell into it, closed my eyes, head in my hands, and tried to will the train forward quickly, to make up for the lost time.

"Suck it up," I thought. "Just get on the plane. If I get to Boston tonight, then I'll make it to the start line. If I get to the start line, I'll make it to the finish."

Walking through O'Hare was painfully slow, literally. I nearly fell twice due to thigh cramps that caused my legs to seize up. Glad for my TSA pre-check status, I negotiated security with little trouble and my gate was blessedly close to the checkpoint. The agent reviewing my ID, vaccination card, and boarding pass was pleasant and wanted to chat about the marathon, but I had to be short with her; I had precious little time left. Shuffling toward the gate, I was anxiously aware of the flight attendants studying my progress.

One of them spoke, "Are you Joseph?" The use of my given name felt ominous. That usually spelled trouble. I was either holding up the show or something worse was going on.

They were probably within a few minutes of giving away my seat. That day, Southwest had some major network disruption that canceled a number of their flights to Boston, thus many travelers were attempting to rebook through United. I suspected that they were coveting my seat. But I made it in time—the flight personnel let me board the plane.

I collapsed into my seat, body aching, and mind muddled. "That went well," I thought.

Getting on the plane was a huge relief but I was not yet out of the woods. In the next 17 hours I had to get back to my Boston Airbnb, hydrate and fuel my body, sleep, and update my blog before changing into a fresh running kit in time to make the 9:15 am shuttle bus to the starting line in Hopkinton. I hoped that my leg cramps would die down by the time I got to the start.

Chicago wasn't easy by a long stretch nor was it painless. But I expected that. The bottom line: my third marathon was in the books, and I was on track to run my fourth in Boston. With only two more left afterward, I felt pretty good about my chances.

How do you like them apples, Parkinson's?

2

A Mystery

Parkinson's disease (PD) is an enigma. What is known is that the neurons in an area of the human midbrain, called the substantia nigra, become impaired and die. The substantia nigra neurons are dopaminergic; that is, they are capable of making dopamine, a neurotransmitter essential for managing mobility and other motor functions. When they die, their dopamine production stops, which causes disruption to muscle movement systems. As of yet, there's no cure. There isn't even a well understood cause.[1,2,3]

Diagnosis is murky as well. To many a casual observer the telltale sign is a tremor, which may affect the fingers, hands, or limbs, but early in the disease the tremors may be subtle or nonexistent. Absent of tremors, a PD sufferer will notice difficulty with balance, strength, and coordination as well as rigidity of movement.[4,5]

Parkinson's typically strikes when the patient is 50 years old or older. It's easy to dismiss early symptoms, as I did, as nothing more than age taking its course. But a skilled neurologist will observe these symptoms, ask some probing questions, push and poke the patient through a series of evaluations to assess motor functions and then likely prescribe medication (typically Sinemet, the brand name for a combination of the generic drugs levodopa and carbidopa, although there are other medications that may be prescribed).[6] Often the acid test is that if the meds help then the patient has PD.

But there's this thing about Parkinson's disease—even as the medications help, the disease continues to progress. Medicating with Sinemet is a dopamine replacement therapy. Nerve cells use the levodopa in Sinemet to make dopamine, which replenishes some of the lost supply.[7] However, levodopa doesn't revive any of the dead neurons nor does it prevent the death of the remaining healthy ones. Without a cure or, alternatively, a therapy that prevents further neuron death, levodopa dosage must increase to compensate for the widening dopamine deficit. At some point, levodopa no longer provides comfort to the patient, as the increased dosage amplifies the side effects that will eventually overshadow the benefits.[8]

The reduction in effectiveness of levodopa has led many patients, and some physicians, to conclude that it's efficacy can be "used up" in a few years and therefore it should be avoided or, perhaps, its usage delayed for as long as possible. This view, though, has been debunked.[9] The lessened impact of levodopa over time is simply a consequence of the progression of Parkinson's (see Chapter 7, Clues). As it stands now, levodopa is the gold standard for PD treatment, and it provides the best quality of life for those suffering from the disease.[10]

As the medications become less effective, tremors increase in severity and the movement, balance, and coordination challenges become onerous. Patients don't die of PD. They live with it and, until a cure is found, they die with it. Their lives are forever changed. Independence can no longer be taken for granted because patients will need assistance to perform essential tasks. Some beloved activities are no longer possible. No one can say when the burden will become insufferable. The disease's progression defies prediction—it could be 10 years, maybe five, or perhaps one. But it's likely to happen before the patient is ready for it. *Parkies need to live while the living is good.*

In late 2017, I found out that two of my older siblings were living with Parkinson's having been diagnosed a few years earlier. It was news to me at the time; however, it's common for the newly diagnosed to keep such information private. My father, who passed away in 2012, also had PD and may have been suffering for decades without acknowledging it to himself or to others.

By about 2014, I'd already noticed my own issues. I've been an avid soccer player since high school and recently my ball-handling skills had deteriorated to the point where I'd botch many routine plays. One time on a family ski trip, I fell downloading from a chairlift. While skiers coming off the next chair deftly skied around me, I struggled to stand up and simply could not without the help of the lift operator.

Irrespective of athletic pursuits, at times my legs felt strangely stiff as if I was walking in the shallow end of a pool. I'd stumble often and falls were not uncommon. Online symptom sleuthing suggested PD but I didn't immediately act on this because, somehow, I concluded that nothing could be done about it. However, the news about the prevalence of PD in my family convinced me to see a doctor. That was early 2018 when I was a month shy of turning 57.

The neurologist confirmed that I had Parkinson's. Ironically, I was at ease with the diagnosis. Relieved, in fact. I'm aware that this is not how such news is usually received, but it seemed a better outcome than being told that I was just getting old. In retrospect, it was probably more nuanced than that. I'm an engineer; we try to be rational and analytical. Calm and collected is how I deal with most things. Having an actual diagnosis for the issues I'd been dealing with felt like a bonus.

I was wrong in my earlier assessment of futility. Something *can* be done about PD. My neurologist prescribed Sinemet and immediately my symptoms improved. A tremor in my right arm grew silent, and I was no longer on the verge of falling whenever I walked. Within a month I was playing soccer with skills I thought I'd lost for good five years before.

My neurologist had more good news for me. She said that one of the most effective therapies for PD was vigorous exercise.[11]

Say what, now?

Vigorous exercise is a lifelong passion of mine. I've always worked out: running, bicycling, swimming, triathlons, soccer, ultimate frisbee, hiking, etc. If she had said that the only worthwhile therapies were learning a foreign language or developing perfect pitch, I'd be crestfallen (albeit outwardly stoic). But I had no problem at all with doubling down on exercise. What luck!

~◌⟁⟁◌~

I'm at a loss to explain the good fortune that I've enjoyed during my life. Overall, I feel as if circumstances tend to go in my favor and I have very little, if anything, to complain about. It's not because I always make good decisions. Far from it. I'm quite capable of being boneheaded.

It's like what Geoffrey Rush's character says early on in *Shakespeare in Love*. "Strangely enough it all turns out well," he explains. "I don't know. It's a mystery."

Here are a few highlights:

When I was very young, maybe 10 or 11, I was reading on the couch in our living room when my mother called for me from the kitchen. When I got there, Mom wasn't able to say why she called for me. Just then, there was a loud crash in the living room. The noise was from a huge chunk of plaster that had fallen from the ceiling and had landed on the couch where I'd been sitting only moments before. Apparently, the plaster had lost its grip on the ceiling due to water leakage from the bathroom above. It's hard to say what would have happened had I not been called away. Concussion, maybe. A headache, at least. Perhaps worse. A mother's love for her child coupled with a display of uncanny intuition spared me from those outcomes.

I did well enough in high school to develop touches of arrogance and entitlement. When it came time to apply for university, I don't remember getting much guidance in the selection process. Either my parents figured I didn't need the help or, more likely, didn't want it. When I look back on that time, I marvel at my ignorance in deciding to apply to only one university. Who does that? What if I wasn't accepted? Fortunately, I got into that one school and MIT (Massachusetts Institute of Technology) worked out well for me.

I was raised on Long Island in New York State while my wife, Lynn, grew up 3,000 miles away in Washington near Seattle. The odds of us ever meeting were slim. Yet, we both studied engineering and graduated to jobs with Hewlett-Packard in Santa Rosa, California.

I met Lynn on her first day. Several of us were eating lunch in the cafeteria when she made a cute, nerdy joke that busted up the table. I was taken—OK, smitten—by her sense of humor and confidence in front of a crowd of engineers she hardly knew. Although it took me more than a year of cluelessness to get around to commitment, that joke portended a future together. Yes, I eventually acted on the premonition, but it was dumb luck to be seated at that lunch table.

Unseen forces with a penchant for influencing human lives are not so rare in art and nature. I'm thinking of the "Under Toad" and its omnipresent foreboding in John Irving's *The World According to Garp*, and "Hangman" snatching words from Jason's stuttering tongue in David Mitchell's *Black Swan Green*. There's also Adam Smith's invisible hand of the free marketplace. And gravity and magnetism, for that matter. Something like this may be going on in my life but in a patently benevolent way. Who knows?

I have plenty of additional examples.

Lynn and I have a son, Aidan, who has the gift of putting people at ease with his humor and thoughtfulness. Aidan tolerated having his dad coach him throughout his Little League and most of his soccer seasons. Our daughter, Kinsey, had little interest in team sports. She did, however, demonstrate early wizardry in the kitchen. With her, I had the thrill of making the family dinner together every Sunday night since she was about 10 years old.

In 1997, during a rare lull in the torrid Palo Alto housing market, we found and bought the house where we raised Kinsey and Aidan. Nowhere in its listing, though, was there any indication that the neighborhood we'd move into was one where we'd thrive amongst other nurturing families who were destined to be our lifelong friends.

The invisible hand that helped to guide my family and my personal life also reached into my profession.

Mine was not a typical career of steady advancement within a single specialty. It was more like a random walk through some of the core technologies of Silicon Valley: semiconductors, disk drives, optics, lasers, and LIDAR. During one stretch of 13 years, through a series of start-ups, acquisitions, and spin-offs combined with impressive adaptability of my coworkers and our physical plant, I was employed at five different companies without so much as a change to my work address or my desk phone number. Yet with all that boom, bust, and upheaval over the course of three decades, I managed a modest amount of success and stayed gainfully employed without interruption. Thus, my family was always provided for.

When the inevitable layoffs finally did come toward the end of my work life, they happened when I was working at crappy, soul-sucking jobs and thanks to the Valley's caution over its tacit ageism, they were accompanied by sizable payoffs in exchange for my promise not to sue for wrongful termination. All in all, I feel that I came out ahead.

I'm not claiming divine supervision. As an agnostic, I can't believe that any deity would have the least bit of interest in my affairs. Yet, somehow, good fortune and I have become frequent companions.

A Parkinson's diagnosis, however, is life altering. It's justifiable to presume that my luck had changed for the worse. Yet, I can't say that this has been the case so far.

That's not to say that I welcomed Parkinson's. No one in their right mind would join this club. But when faced with a relentless, progressive neurological disease it does little good to bemoan the situation and live in fear of it. If it really is incurable, what is there to lose? Why not run with it, embrace the experience, adapt, and see how it turns out?

At the time of my diagnosis, Lynn and I had recently become empty-nesters and were looking to shake things up anyway. We already had a plan in place to retire and move to Seattle near where she had grown up. PD gave us a reason to get on with it. We thought that this was a great opportunity to set up camp, relax, and relish the damp grandeur of the Pacific Northwest.

Retirement afforded me the time to step up the exercise. Initially, I planned to focus on biking expecting that it would help with my balance issues. I also considered turning my attention to kayaking given that our home was within a few steps of a convenient Puget Sound beach. So many islands and vistas to explore! However, the climate of the Pacific Northwest eventually shoved me in a different direction. Curiously, I found that I actually enjoyed running in the rain. Truth be told, I sweat so heavily when I run that staying dry is never an option for me anyway.

Running turned out to be more than mere therapy. It's been a game changer.

3

Learning to Run

Before the Parkinson's diagnosis, my typical run would be three to five miles and I'd do an occasional 5K or 10K road race[1] when the competitive spirit moved me. Motivated by a desire to manage my new disorder and with an abundance of retirement time on my hands, however, I thought I'd try some longer distances.

I ran my first half marathon in May 2019, at age 58, with the goal of finishing in 1 hour 55 minutes. I figured that if the half went well, I would take on a full marathon. I bested my goal in that half marathon by nearly three minutes—it was time to take aim at a full marathon.

My marathon goal was to BQ; that is, to have a finish time fast enough to meet the qualifying standard for the prestigious Boston Marathon. Qualifying to enter Boston is the goal of many a runner. I decided to shoot for the 2021 race when I would be 60, so the BQ standard for me, set by the race's administrator, the Boston Athletic Association (BAA), was 3:50:00.[2] For my qualifying race, I entered the California International Marathon (CIM) held in Sacramento on December 8, 2019. I chose CIM because, historically, a high percentage of its runners qualify for Boston.

This is when things got more serious. Despite all the running I'd done up until then, I was ignorant of what it takes to run a full marathon. I was also ignorant of proper technique for running long distances. Hence, at the advanced age of 58 it was finally time for me to learn how to run.

It's been said that a full marathon is four times as hard as a half. My daughter, Kinsey, said that to me. Before she left for college, Kinsey and I would run 10Ks and triathlons together. In college, she joined a running club and by graduation she had already bagged two marathons, including Boston. My running lessons often began as conversations with her after which I'd follow up with internet research to better understand what she said.

As my weekly mileage grew, I went through a lot of supplies, which I obtained from my local running store, West Seattle Runner (WSR). The owners, Tim and Lori McConnell, are not only passionate about running, they really impressed me with their customer service and dedication to the West Seattle community. So, on one of my visits to WSR, when I saw a "Help Wanted" sign out front, the urge to apply for the job was strong. I worked there for two years beginning in October 2019.

Like an immersive language program, a running store provides the environment for a newbie marathoner to absorb all there is to know about running. Tim and Lori and their store manager, Ferguson Mitchell, got me up to speed very quickly.

It might appear as if this was my plan all along. It wasn't. I just really liked the store and thought I should get out of the house and interact with people occasionally. Or maybe it was that invisible hand doing its thing again? I'll never know. That's just one of the things about invisibility—*you never know.*

Here's a brief review of my running indoctrination with some of my own prejudices tossed in:

Training Plan

Over the years I have spoken to some would-be marathoners who didn't make it to the start line because they got injured during training. That's a significant takeaway. Injuries are common among all runners but especially so with marathoners. Any training plan worthy of a neophyte must be designed to avoid injury.

For CIM, I used a 16-week training plan crafted by *Runner's World* (RW) that I believe is based on Jack Daniels' (the coach, not the distiller) running formula.[3] I don't recall exactly why I chose this one but most likely it was because the source was reputable and downloading it was free.

Here are some features of the training plan:

- The plan starts off at a total of 31 miles in the first week. Weekly mileage totals increase gradually, typically by less than 10% per week until week 13 and then taper off for the final three weeks of the plan. Tapering ensures that the body is adequately rested heading into race day.
- Nearly half of the miles are run slowly; that is, one to two minutes slower than the runner's goal pace for race day. For example, I wanted to finish CIM in 3:45:00,

implying a race pace of 8 minutes 35 seconds (8:35) per mile. For these slow training sessions then, my target pace was about 9:30 to 10:30 per mile.

- Faster-paced training sessions include tempo, intervals, and hill repeats, which are all intended to develop speed and strength. *RW* also has a website that provides the suggested paces for all these training sessions that are calculated from the runner's targeted marathon finish time.[4]
- A single long run is planned for each week and is one of the slow-paced runs. My plan's long runs started at 9 miles and eventually ramped up to 21 miles. Long runs are intended to build endurance and injury is avoided by running them slowly.
- Rest days are included in the plan. I chose to run five days each week while resting the other two days.

Rest

I was relieved to find that nowadays experts advise runners to include rest days into their schedule to allow the body to repair damage caused by the training. Perhaps my strongest feature as a runner is that I'm retired; it allows me to take a post-workout nap whenever I need it, which is most days. I'm thoroughly impressed by marathoners with full-time responsibilities who manage to fit in their training despite having schedules that don't allow for any spontaneous downtime.

Protection From Mechanical Abuse

From my engineering days I knew about the damage that a harsh environment can do to a mechanical assembly. I used to build microelectronic and optoelectronic devices. To protect them from premature death, we'd isolate them from shocks and vibrations using absorbing materials and we'd take pains to assemble the device as securely as possible so that violent shaking wouldn't spontaneously disassemble them.

It must be that the human body reacts analogously to the running environment. Forces up to three times the runner's weight are generated with each foot strike. A reasonable approach toward isolating the body from these forces is to start at the bottom. I wear the thickly cushioned running shoes from HOKA. Walking in these shoes can be described as like walking on clouds or marshmallows. The force generated by each foot strike is absorbed by the shoe rather than by my body.

For securing my leg muscles, I use compression shorts and knee-high compression socks. To be honest, I've been wearing compression stockings during all waking hours since my early 40s because of a bad case of varicose veins. The compression works together with the muscles of the lower leg to return deoxygenated blood back to the heart.

Besides improving circulation, the compression protects the legs from vibrational stresses that can cause micro-tears in the muscle fibers.

Long distances used to mess up my legs. Muscle strains and aches were very common. But these injuries have been much more rare since I started wearing HOKA's and compression clothing.

I'm a scientist. OK, fine, an engineer then. Either way, I'm aware that I haven't done a thorough experimental validation of my faith in either cushioning or compression. Proper experimental design, however, is a serious challenge. For example, the accepted gold standard of validation is the randomized double-blind experiment comparing the treatment to a placebo, which is believed to have no relevant efficacy or is being used as a control. If the treatment performs better than the placebo, then the treatment has been validated.

But how could a double-blind experiment be performed for this hypothesis? Have someone dress me in shoes, shorts, and socks in such a way that neither of us are aware of what I'm running in? The mind boggles.

In fairness, then, this practice of mine for shoes and apparel may be a placebo. And I'm OK with that because I'm a big believer in the placebo effect. It's very powerful. It's the most universally accepted medical treatment for a wide range of ailments. That's why when Big Pharma tries to put out a new drug, if they want the FDA to approve it, then they have to prove it works better than green M&M's. Turns out, green M&M's are hard to beat.

This is one example of why running, much like all of human medicine, is as much an art as it is a science. Experience and experimentation lead to an array of best practices that work for many runners. For the individual runner, it's a matter of trying them and discarding those that are unhelpful or unappealing.

I'm sticking with HOKA's and compression apparel unless and until something breaks. And, speaking of art, I like my socks to be colorful because of the positive feedback I get from friends and passers-by. I wear a variety of colors but my preference for race day is hot pink. Not everyone can pull that off, but I've yet to hear any complaints.

Knee-high compression socks can be a bear to put on. A fair bit of finger strength and mechanical leverage is needed to get them over the heel. As I age and my fingers weaken, I may need to invent some type of application tool if I'm to continue wearing them.

Form

Long distance running is not at all like the explosive, muscular sprints of soccer or other similar sports. Nowadays, soccer tends to mess up my calf muscles and my hamstrings, compression clothing notwithstanding. With longer distances there's a whole new set of injuries to contend with. Many of these are mitigated by using the proper running form.

There are many sources of running information on the internet. One that I've enjoyed for its simplicity and clarity is McMillan Running.[5]

Running can be thought of as a "controlled fall." The torso is tall with a slight lean to create the falling-forward momentum (*posture*). Legs cycle rapidly with each step timed to keep the center of mass moving forward rather than crashing into the ground (*cadence*). And with each stride the foot comes down directly beneath the center of mass (*foot strike*).

As is the case with all sports, inefficiency is to be avoided. I classify inefficiency in running form into two broad categories: 1) wasted motion that doesn't contribute to moving the runner forward and 2) motion that puts the runner at risk of injury. There's more to it, but I would assert that getting a solid grasp of these three qualities—posture, cadence, and foot strike—has gotten me most of the way there.[6]

> *Posture:* Good running posture mitigates much of the inefficiency of wasted motion. Runners should stand tall with a slight forward lean at the ankles that sets off the controlled fall.
>
> When runners slouch in the torso or sag at the hips the legs get crammed into a tighter vertical space. To make room for the legs to swing through their arc, extra effort is needed to drive the body's center of mass upward. This

vertical motion doesn't contribute to moving the runner forward and thus represents a wasteful expense of energy.

Running tall also helps keep a runner's lower legs straight up with less side-to-side motion and less bending laterally at the knee, both of which are wasteful.

Similarly, a tall posture discourages arm swing that crosses the midline of the body out in front of the runner. That's a sideways motion that doesn't help move the body forward.

Cadence: The force generated with each foot fall can do a lot of damage to the runner if not managed. Cadence, or the number of steps taken per minute (spm), effects this force. Quick, light steps produce less impact stress than long, heavier ones and therefore fatigue is reduced as is the potential for injury.

At the 1984 Olympics, legendary running coach Jack Daniels measured the cadence of elite runners, and they all came in at about 180 spm. With this observation, somehow 180 spm became the cadence gold standard. One way to match that cadence is by having the runner listen to songs that race along at 180 beats per minute (bpm) and time his stride to match the beat. Playlists of 180 bpm songs are available on the internet. For example, just about any *Ramones* song will do.

But the 180 spm as a gold standard is questionable given the highly filtered sampling of only elite runners.[7] McMillan Running states that the ideal cadence varies depending on the runner and is likely to be in the range of 170-190 spm.[8]

It's often suggested that a runner should maintain the ideal cadence whether running slow or fast, but I'm not so sure. Experience dictates to me that a higher cadence means a faster pace. When at my top speed my cadence is about 175 spm but I'm not able to keep that up for very long. For the hours-long stretch of a marathon, I'm content to coast along at 165 spm.

Foot Strike: A common error when running long-distance is overstriding wherein the foot strikes the ground too far in front of the body's center of mass. It's especially prevalent when a runner tries to run faster by striding out with her steps thrown farther out in front. This is a classic cause of knee pain.

Rather, the runner should always have their feet land directly below them in line with their center of mass. A misaligned center of mass generates torque that wrenches the knee thus causing pain. When striding out, the foot should continue to land in the same place but with the legs pushed out longer behind the runner.

I once evaluated the gait of a runner who was also a dancer complaining of knee pain. She had this long, absolutely beautiful stride, each of which looked like an elegant *grand jeté*. Fantastic for a dancer but painful for a runner—slow cadence with a landing way out in front of the center of mass. To run without pain, she would have to abandon that style.

These three qualities are not independent. Proper execution of one of them can pull others in line. For example, a rapid cadence (with a shorter stride) helps with foot strike because if the feet are moving quickly enough, they won't have enough time to get into an overstriding position.

It's relatively straightforward to get these elements under control when fresh into a run. However, and this is a big problem of mine that I continue to work on, as the miles pile up, form suffers. It can be a nasty feedback cycle; for example, fatigue induces a drop in cadence which, when unchecked, increases fatigue and drops cadence further.

Runners notoriously pay inadequate attention to muscle development in the hips, butt, and core. When these poorly developed muscles tire and weaken on long runs, posture suffers, efficiency drops, and risk of injury increases.

It's a maintenance task that must be tended to throughout a long run and especially during the latter half of it. It's very common for me to feel more jarring on my body with each step as the miles pile up. Eventually, I'll clue in and force the necessary tweaks—stand up straight, don't slouch, lift up your hips, pick up the cadence, don't over stride, you got this.

Fueling

The thought of fueling during a marathon was a novelty to me. My strategy had always been to run, bike, play soccer, etc. on an empty stomach, because, well, I don't know why. Like every other exercise nut in the world, I knew that runners carbo load before races. But I never knew much about the details until now.

Carbo loading made the scene in the late 1960s when a Swedish physiologist, Gunvar Ahlborg, worked out the role that glycogen plays in the performance of endurance athletes.[9,10,11]

Running a marathon requires a lot of fuel. Due to how rapidly carbohydrates can mobilize, they're the body's fuel of choice for race day. Glucose, the simple sugar studied during the photosynthesis section of high school biology class, is the carb that actually powers a cell. Glycogen is just a large number of glucose molecules bonded together in a way that makes it easy for the body to separate them for use wherever and whenever they're needed.

The human body can store about 600 grams of glycogen. Most of it, about 500 grams, is stored in the muscle cells and nearly all the rest of it is stored in the liver. A tiny bit hides out in the brain.

That level of glycogen will fuel a runner somewhere between 90 minutes to 2 hours. When emptied of glycogen the runner hits the proverbial wall, the ability and desire to continue ebbs, and the runner questions why she ever wanted to run a marathon in the first place.

It's worse when the runner's glycogen storage is not full to begin with. In this case, the crash can happen much sooner. Carbo loading, when done properly, allows the runner to start the race with a full glycogen tank.

Is a full glycogen tank enough? No.

Runners, even the elites who finish a marathon in about two hours, need to eat all through the race. It's generally accepted that a runner needs to consume 30 to 60 grams of carbohydrates per hour.

This keeps the glucose available to cells via the bloodstream thus slowing the burn rate of the stored glycogen.

Just about any carb will do (e.g., cookies, peanut butter sandwiches, raw fruit, dried fruit, jellybeans, etc.), but there are some practical considerations to contend with when eating while running a marathon. For example, a dry carb eaten on the go can be uncomfortable and is potentially a choking hazard. A runner will want to wash the food down with water just like at any meal, so there needs to be a water source handy. The runner can carry water or obtain some at an aid station along the race route. Alternatively, carbs that come in a liquid form are easier to consume and faster to digest so that they get to the muscles more quickly than do dry carbs.

Also, it's best if the food doesn't make the runner sick. How do you run a marathon with an upset stomach? Or, to use the broader terminology that some runners prefer, how do you run when under GI (gastrointestinal) distress? Runners choose to practice eating their preferred carbs on training runs so that there are no uncomfortable surprises on race day.

Unsurprisingly, there are many prepackaged, carb-laced products available to meet the fueling needs of runners (e.g., gooey, frosting-like gels; solid gels; packaged nut butters; packaged maple syrup; etc.). Most ubiquitous are the gooey gels, which don't work for me. Not that I've ever tried them. They just make me queasy thinking about sucking them down during a run.

I like to eat Clif Bloks on long runs and races because they're like candy, and I can wrap my mind around candy. These energy chews come in packages containing six cubes, and I will down three of them every three miles. That works out to 90 calories and 23 grams of carbs every 25 to 30 minutes. I do need water to wash them down which is fine because I like to wear a hydration vest when I do long distances and I planned for that at CIM.

I've also tried Maurten Gels as an alternative to Clif Bloks. The carbs in Maurten are bound up in a hydrogel, which, according to the manufacturer, protects them from digestion in the stomach so they go right to the intestines where the digestion is more efficient. Also, there's a lot of water in the hydrogel so there's no need for additional water to wash it down. Maurten products are very popular with elite runners these days.

Hydration, on the other hand, has always made perfect sense to me. Sweat, get thirsty, drink water. Got it. I remember when growing up there would be the occasional story of a football player who died from dehydration/heat stroke at practice when the temperature was in the 80s or higher. I knew firsthand how coaches in those days thought that it was a sign of weakness for a player to request water on hot days. Sadly, high school sports-related dehydration deaths still occur from time to time.

There's more to hydration science than just water.

Researchers at the University of Florida were urged by the school's head football coach to study how to help athletes replace fluids lost from sweating. The result was Gatorade, which debuted in 1965.[12]

The researchers discovered that sweat contains a lot of ions, primarily sodium ($Na+$), an element in salt ($NaCl$), which is why sweat tastes salty. There are also ions of potassium, chloride, and calcium, among others. Nowadays, when used in the context of sports nutrition, these ions are called electrolytes.

The thinking was that along with water, the body needed to have the electrolytes replenished for optimum performance. Therefore, they mixed up some electrolytes with water and sugar, called it Gatorade, and gave it to the football team during practice and games to generally positive reviews.

Classic double-blind experimental opportunity missed. Who knows how well a placebo would have done?

Yet, electrolyte replenishment is here to stay and there is scientific basis to support its validity.[13] Water flows into or out of cells based on the relative concentrations of ions within and surrounding them.

It's like when seasoning steak or chicken by sprinkling it with salt causing a higher concentration of salt on the outside of the meat's cells than on the inside. That imbalance draws water out of the meat to collect on the surface. Conversely, a lower concentration of ions outside of cells than on the inside pulls water into them. For a runner, ideally the system is in equilibrium—water stays put flowing neither into nor out of the cell—because net water flow in either direction across the cell membrane is problematic and can lead to dehydration and other conditions.

Therefore, it's not enough to simply drink water. To avoid dehydration, the electrolytes must be replaced as well to maintain the ion balance across the cell membrane. A runner would do well to keep this in mind during the heat of competition. Every hour, a runner will need to drink three-quarters of a liter of water while taking in 600 mg of sodium.

As is the case with nutrition, there are many hydration products for athletes to choose from. Some, like Gatorade, include sugar so that carb replacement takes place at the same time as hydration.

There are other products, however, with very little sugar. They address the possibility that the runner may not always want or need carbs when rehydrating. This might be the case for contests of less than one hour where glycogen replacement is not necessary.

I sweat a lot when I run thanks to Parkinson's. Excessive sweating is one of many PD symptoms. I prefer to hydrate with a product having few calories because I want to be able to add more electrolytes to the stew without having to take on more carbs. I typically use Nuun, which has 300 mg of sodium in each tablet.

For CIM, I planned to wear the hydration pack having four Nuun tablets dissolved in two liters of water. That's a total of 1,200 mg of sodium in solution with the water. I get another 1,150 mg in the 24 Clif Bloks I eat during the race. Even that's not enough for me so I would down some more electrolyte drinks at the aid stations provided on the course.

Inadequate hydration leads to muscle cramps. Parkinson's disease also features muscle cramps. Muscle cramps, unsurprisingly then, are a big issue for me and it's important to get the hydration right. I also have found that the cramps are persistent thus making for a long recovery period. To rid my body of them, I must drink electrolyte-laced water for several hours after a long run.

The carbs, water, and electrolytes take care of the on-course fueling needs and, as mentioned, they're also eaten when not running. The other part of the mix is protein. Protein is required for tissue repair during recovery. There's a rule of thumb that runners should eat in a 4:1 carbs to protein ratio right after a race and after training sessions to optimize the body's ability to repair the damage that has been done.

I don't claim to be an expert in all things regarding marathon running. But this concise synopsis worked well enough for me.

4

Escalating Goals

It was a perfect day for a race at the 2019 California International Marathon (CIM). A little bit of rain but otherwise low humidity and the temperature was about 50 degrees. But the thrilling part was the spectator support. I had never run such a large race and I was surprised to see so many people lining the route shouting support to all the strangers passing by. I could get used to this.

I did manage to BQ but not by much—I finished in 3:49:25.

Some clarification of the BQ is in order. Achieving a BQ during the qualification period for the Boston Marathon allows the runner to apply to enter the race. However, there are nearly always more applicants than the maximum allowable field size (typically 30,000 runners), so an application alone is not sufficient. To actually gain entry into the race it's necessary to beat the relevant qualifying standard by at least the cutoff time (the larger the number of excess applicants, the longer the cutoff time). The length of the cutoff time is set by the BAA and is used to trim the applicant pool down to the field size limit and ensures that only the fastest runners earn a race bib.

This works for the BAA but is a nuisance for runners. When runners line up for their qualification race, they won't know how much faster than their standard they need to be because the cutoff time is not determined until the BAA counts the number of applicants during the registration period. Runners therefore must hedge their bets. A reasonable guess may be to aim at beating their standard by 5-10 minutes. That's why my target for CIM was to finish under 3:45. I figured that a five-minute cutoff margin would be sufficient.

I missed the target, and my cutoff margin was only 35 seconds. By the CIM race day the cutoff time for the 2020 Boston Marathon had already been set at 1 minute 39 seconds and demand for running in Boston year over year nearly always increases as does the cutoff time. For the 2021 race, the one I planned to run, surely the cutoff time would be longer than 35 seconds.

So, my plan was to enter another marathon or two in 2020. I needed another shot at finishing under 3:45 thereby providing the cutoff margin I would need to earn a Boston bib.

But what about after Boston? What would be my next goal?

That's when I learned of the Abbott World Marathon Majors.[1] Abbott WMM celebrates runners of all stripes who complete all six of the Marathon Majors: Tokyo, Boston, London, Berlin, Chicago, and New York City. A runner earns a WMM Star for each of the Majors that they run. Upon finishing the sixth, the runner is awarded the Six Star Medal and with it the corresponding bragging rights.

According to the Abbott WMM website in December 2019, more than 6,000 runners had completed the series. Often it took years to finish all six. If they could manage to enter and train for any of them at all, it may only be one or two of the races each year. For people with full-time responsibilities, doing even one Major per year can be impossible so there may be many seemingly idle years before the Six Star Medal is earned.

A few runners, less than 100,[2] achieved the feat in a single calendar year. That spoke to me. As a Parkie I couldn't be sure how many years of distance running I had left in me. As a retiree, though, I had the free time needed to devote to the training and the travel required to get them all done in a single year if that year was not too far in the future. Perfect. I set my goal to run all six of the Majors in 2021. Normally this meant running Tokyo, Boston, and London in the spring and the rest of them in the fall.

I set this goal at the end of 2019 not knowing that the world was on the brink of a wholesale calamity.

The coronavirus pandemic disrupted the World Marathon Majors along with everything else going on across the globe. COVID-19 had an immediate effect on these races. The outbreak started in China in mid-December 2019, near enough in time and place to the Tokyo Marathon scheduled for March 1, 2020, that race directors acted promptly to protect the health and safety of runners and spectators. Field size, originally set at nearly 37,500 runners, was reduced to only 200 or so elite athletes. The one million spectators typically lining the course were actively discouraged from attending.

Similarly, London downsized its field to allow only elite runners and prohibited spectators. Normally held on the streets of London from Greenwich to Buckingham Palace, the 2020 course was redrawn as multiple laps around St. James Park.

All the other Majors were canceled outright.

As the pandemic raged, the fate of the 2021 Majors was uncertain. Toward the end of 2020, newly developed vaccines brought hope for 2021 although too late for the races traditionally held in the spring. They would be rescheduled for the fall.

By the end of 2020, the plan for the following year took shape. Berlin, Chicago, and New York City had already secured their dates (September 26, October 10, and November 7, respectively). London and Tokyo chose to work within this envelope with London opting for October 3 and Tokyo selecting October 17.

Five marathons in six weeks. Ouch! My goal had gone from challenging to uncertain to absurd in the matter of a few months. Boston had yet to make a scheduling decision, but I figured they'd fit themselves in either before Berlin or on one of the free weekends between Tokyo and New York City. It would be tough, for sure, but I was still game.

Then on January 26, 2021, the Boston Athletic Association announced that they'd hold their marathon on Monday, October 11, the day after Chicago's.

Shit!

The news was disconcerting to put it mildly. Conventional running lore holds that a marathon so wrecks the body that weeks and sometimes months of recovery are necessary. Indeed, after CIM in December 2019 I had to take a break from training that lasted deep into January.

Six marathons in six weeks across three continents with two of them held on consecutive days. Very little time for recovery.

Was it about time to reassess my goals? Maybe reschedule for 2022?

No.

Goals are insidious. Once entrenched they are hard to dislodge even when supporting assumptions are changed drastically. Like when the Black Knight continues to refuse Arthur's passage despite losing all his limbs to the good King.[3] Yes, it's lunacy to insist that the battle is not already lost, but, *see, there was this goal.*

Obstinance can be a good thing. Ambitious objectives pursued relentlessly may be at worst foolishly heroic whereas capitulation to shabby, unforeseen circumstances feels like failure accepted all too readily.

Was I obsessed with my goal? Yeah, I suppose so. But I've learned that this isn't uncommon among people who have Parkinson's disease. There are many examples of Parkies challenging themselves with athletic endeavors better suited to the young and able. Time is not on our side; we can't be certain when it will be our last opportunity to say, *"Take that, Parkinson's, and shove it!"*

I thought a lot about the challenge of running six marathons stuffed into those six weeks. I was certain that my friends and family would call me out for the nuttiness of the enterprise. I was willing to go for it on faith but to really convince myself and others that it was possible, I needed a coherent plan for success. I did what we engineers do—I studied the problem, challenged assumptions, and called upon my substantial reserves of pigheadedness. With that a kernel of a strategy took shape.

Consider the training. I had newly experienced that marathon training is just as hard if not harder than the race itself. Get through the training without injury and the race itself may feel like a walk in the park.

Also, let's consider that fixture of most training plans—the weekly long run. Long runs are done at a pace one to two minutes slower than the target race pace. The idea is to train one's body to be on the move for three to four hours as a way to build the endurance required while the slower pace minimizes the chance of injury.

Furthermore, conventional wisdom notwithstanding, it's the attempt at a personal record (PR) that devastates the body. And elites who are going for the win don't race again the next week, or even the next month, because at that level of performance a runner needs rest. The harder the beat down the longer the recuperation time.

Therefore, here's the gist. Casting aside aspirations of a podium finish (as if) or even a PR, why not just train as if it's for the last marathon in New York City and then consider the rest of the races as weekly long runs that just happen to be 26.2

miles long? Do the long, slow run thing if that's what it takes to recover in time for the next week's race.

As viewed through this lens, the compressed schedule of these marathons is an advantage. There'd be only one training cycle rather than six. If the goal is to complete all six Majors in a single year, well then, how convenient! I had no doubt that others had figured this out and that I would have company.

I could work with this. But then there's still that pesky Boston Marathon the day after Chicago giving me less than 24 hours to recover. What's the plan for that one, smart guy?

Screw your courage to the sticking place.

It turns out that running marathons on consecutive days is a thing now, and it's become more popular perhaps due to the pandemic cancellation of so many in-person races forcing runners to turn to novel solo competitive outlets. One extreme example: In 2020, Alyssa Clark ran 95 consecutive daily marathons. (Ironically, it was a nonfatal bout with COVID-19 that ended her streak.)

Diehards running back-to-back marathons are not so rare. Understandably, the folks who do such things have no qualms about posting in detail about their strategies on social media. It can be done, there's a body of internet literature describing how to do it, and I had the better part of nine months to apply it to my situation.

My traveling to all these races meant that I would be spending a lot of time in the air, and I regretted the substantial carbon footprint involved. I actually wondered whether someone like Greta Thunberg would call me out for my selfishness. I spent some time researching other less climate-damaging transportation options. Take the train between Chicago and Boston? Cargo ship travel to Europe? Arguably less planet impactful but no other option met my schedule. It seemed the best I could do was to spend some guilt money and so I purchased nearly 55,000 pounds worth of carbon offsets in February.[4] Not a great solution but acceptable.

I must point out that setting this goal and strategizing on how to achieve it took place entirely within my head. From the time I conceived it at the end of 2019 until early in 2021, I kept it to myself as I worked through the details. In other words, while I obsessed, my wife and children were oblivious.

When I finally let them in on the plan in February 2021, it's not surprising that we came at the news from completely different perspectives. While I had a year to totally internalize and justify the adventure with casual nonchalance, they hadn't the opportunity to incorporate all the ramifications. In short, they were blindsided.

My son, Aidan, was worried that I would be putting myself unnecessarily at risk to the coronavirus and to my own stubborn need to achieve. He knew very well what my public declaration of this goal meant. "When you tell others about a plan of yours," he states, "that means you've already decided to do it. There's no turning back for you."

Like Aidan, Kinsey knew that I'd committed myself to the goal. In a way it made perfect sense—her dad always went after the harder challenges. She was worried, though. As a marathoner herself, she was well aware of the risks of running one let alone six of them in six weeks. On top of that there was the COVID-19 risk.

Lynn knew all this and more. She is, and always has been, my primary confidant and advisor. Ever since my PD diagnosis, Lynn has been protective of my well-being. At the same time, she has admired how I've stayed so positive since the diagnosis and how diligently I've focused on my health.

"Joe," she has said, "you've become a running machine."

Yet, this goal made no sense to Lynn and for good reason. In her mind, if the marathons didn't incapacitate me then very likely COVID-19 would. This was just insane! Was it worth the risk? She also feared, justifiably, that it was already too late for her to influence me. She felt powerless to fix this problem that her husband handed to her.

Despite my tendency for stubbornness, I'm not without my merits. In just the last few years I acquiesced to move to Seattle and now Lynn lives in close proximity to her mother and sisters and can visit with them at will. I scored major points for that one. Also, I recognize all the meal planning, grocery shopping, and dinner preparation that she did while the kids were growing up. Now, in retirement, I do all these chores for our household. Lynn has earned the respite. And I diligently prepare coffee for her every morning.

I don't lord all this over her.

Well, I guess, sometimes I do. That's beside the point.

The point is that I've built up some goodwill in our relationship. My plan frightened her, but she listened to my reasons for doing it and to my explanations as to how I'd handle the training, the travel, and other risks that may come up. I don't think that I ever convinced her that any of it made sense but she ultimately accepted it and helped me wherever she could. It's just one more thing I love about her. Parkinson's has added a measure of the inexplicable to our relationship but I can still count on her to support me unconditionally.

Now, how do I enter all these races? After all, one does not simply walk into the Boston Marathon.

⚬ ⬓ ⬒ ⚬

There are several ways to get into each of the WMM:[5]

- Win a place via a lottery held by the race
- Qualify based on meeting the race's time standard
- Obtain entry as part of an international tour package
- Enter as a charity runner

The lottery approach was a bust for me. I missed the lotteries for the international races, New York chose not to hold one for 2021, and Boston never has one.

At registration time my only certified marathon finish was 3:49:25, which met the qualifying standard for 60-year-old men both for Chicago (4:00:00) and Boston (3:50:00) but not for New York City (3:34:00). In the interest of pandemic safety, Boston chose to drop their field size down to 20,000 runners from the usual 30,000. They did this by increasing the cutoff time that was previously stated as 3 minutes 3 seconds to 7 minutes 47 seconds thereby cancelling the entry for 10,000 runners. I missed the new cut by a long shot with my CIM finish time.

The qualification standards for US citizens in the international races are even more aggressive than for the domestic ones, so no help there. Thus, my certified finish time only gets me into Chicago. That's fine, I'll take it.

Interestingly, as it turns out, noncitizens *can* simply walk into the international marathons by booking a ticket with a company specializing in marathon tours (i.e., International Tour Operators or ITOs). The ticket comes with a few nights' stay in the marathon city with like-minded runners, one or more tours of the city, a race bib, and some hand-holding to get to and from the race Expo[6] and the race itself. I went with this for both Berlin and Tokyo.

About Tokyo. On June 17, 2021, five months after believing I had secured a bib for it, in the face of rising COVID-19 fears, race authorities in Tokyo announced that they were restricting the marathon to allow only Japan residents.[7] That sucked. Messed up my goal big time; I resigned myself to achieving at best only five-sixths of my goal. I'll have to defer to some other year to be named later and I'd be race-idle on October 17.

So that leaves the charity approach for London, Boston, and New York City. Nonprofits and other organizations partner with each of the races to secure spots allocated by the race directors for charitable causes. In exchange for a bib, the runner is obligated to raise money for the charity to the tune of a few thousand to more than ten thousand dollars depending on the race and the charity.

Choosing a charitable organization to support was a no-brainer for me. If they would have me, my most logical choice was The Michael J. Fox Foundation for Parkinson's Research.

5

Team Fox

In late 1990, Michael J. Fox (MJF) was at the top of his game and poised to take it to another level when the pinkie finger on his left hand sent him a message.

If he hadn't already been a household name with his work in television (e.g., *Family Ties, The 25,000 Pyramid,* and various guest roles), his budding film career certified it. The breakout *Back to the Future* trilogy was huge and his talents were frequently on display on the big screen worldwide (e.g., *Teen Wolf, Bright Lights, Big City, The Secret of My Success,* etc.).

But the pinkie finger, wiggling uncontrollably, was telling him that he was to enter a new era of his life. The wiggle was a tremor and in 1991 at the age of 29, MJF was diagnosed with young-onset Parkinson's disease.[1]

Afterward, understandably, there was a dark period for him as he dealt with the effects of the disease and the disruption to his livelihood. But then he did a most remarkable thing. He shrugged off his denial, depression, and destructive behavior and pivoted to advocacy using his fame to bring awareness of PD to a wider audience.

In 2000, he created the foundation that bears his name—The Michael J. Fox Foundation for Parkinson's Research (MJFF)—which has since raised over one billion dollars toward seeking a cure for Parkinson's.[2]

Notably, MJF never wanted a large endowment for his foundation. That would send the message that this foundation was in it for the long haul. Quite the opposite, MJFF wants to be irrelevant as soon as possible because irrelevance means that a cure has been found and the job is done.

Thus, the method by which the Foundation allocates funding; the money doesn't sit still for long. It's immediately put to work. MJFF finds the most promising research trends, especially risky ones that Big Pharma isn't inclined to fund, and injects capital into them to accelerate progress.

Before MJFF, PD research was largely fractious, inefficient, and, at times, confoundingly adversarial. MJFF brought focus to the work and 21 years later there's been much progress in the understanding of the disease, including the signature pathologies of the PD brain and the variety of ways by which the disease manifests. As of yet there is still no cure but there is a steady pipeline of new drugs and therapies in clinical trials.[3]

I didn't know much of this when I started on my task of securing race bibs for the 2021 WMM. I was simply matching my quest to an appropriate charity that I could get behind. I've since read all of MJF's books and his story is beyond impressive. Not for nothing, it interests me that we're the same age. He was born three months to the day after I was. Damn him, though, for still looking like the Marty McFly of 1985.

MJF has taken some criticism for being so perennially upbeat and optimistic. But in a recent book, *No Time Like the Future*, he details a very bad year of spinal surgery to remove a paralyzing benign tumor, subsequent rehab, an accidental fall that broke his arm, and yet more rehab, he comes around to the realities of PD for many sufferers. "I can't put a shiny face on this," he writes. "This sucks, and who am I to tell people to be optimistic?"[4]

Still, how does one go about changing the world without a substantial measure of optimism?

I'm one of the lucky ones. My Parkinson's symptoms are, for now at least, relatively mild. There are others not as fortunate and MJFF has provided a means by which I can channel my blessings toward helping other PD sufferers.

MJFF reaches out to the PD community with opportunities to participate in research studies, support groups, and fundraising. Community volunteers who help raise money for MJFF are members of Team Fox. Over 5,500 individuals have raised more than $100 million since 2006.[5] Most Team Fox members host their own events (e.g., golf tournaments, pancake breakfasts, fun runs, etc.) though some support MJFF through participating in endurance events around the world. These include all the World Marathon Majors other than Tokyo.

In researching Team Fox, I came across the name of Associate Director Liz Berger. Her job is to recruit for, plan, and execute on the Team Fox endurance events. I contacted Liz and explained my desire to run all the WMM in 2021. At our first phone call, I was fully prepared with my pitch explaining how I would achieve this goal. But to her credit and to my surprise, she never once expressed anything but support for it. Never did she suggest that this quest was anything but doable. I suspect that she has more than average familiarity with the resolve that Parkies can muster.

Liz immediately got me on Team Fox as a charity runner in the London Marathon. And once Boston and New York City solidified their plans she welcomed me to those races as well.

Liz is one of my heroes at Team Fox. She introduced me to another one, Bill Bucklew. Bill was diagnosed with young-onset PD in 2012 at the age of 43. Among many other adventures, in January 2018, he completed a 2,500-mile cross-country trek from Georgia to San Diego walking the equivalent of two marathons each day. He did this to raise awareness for PD and $100,000 for MJFF.[6]

Bill did a TED Talk about that cross-country journey.[7] In his presentation he revealed that a panel of doctors who evaluated him prior to the trek advised him not to do it given the mobility issues they observed. I cherish his response to that advice. He thought about what it would mean to him if he failed at this effort. He decided that it was "OK to fail," and therefore, full steam ahead.

Bill had entered the 2021 London, Chicago, and New York City Marathons with Team Fox and so we would soon cross paths. And get this: He planned to run London the day after completing his latest challenge, *The Long Walk for Parkinson's*, wherein he'd walk from the northern end of Scotland to London, 670 miles, in 17 days.[8]

On the MJFF website I read up on other Team Fox members with stories similar to Bill's—Bret Parker and Jimmy Choi.

Bret Parker was diagnosed with young-onset PD in 2007 at the age of 38. He kept that diagnosis to himself until 2012 and since then he's been a fundraising juggernaut with over $800,000 raised through Team Fox activities. In 2018, he participated in the World Marathon Challenge wherein athletes run in seven marathons on seven continents in seven days.[9] Makes my goal look like a leisurely stroll to the corner store.

Like Bill, Bret, and MJF, Jimmy Choi was diagnosed with young-onset PD in 2003 at the age of 27. As late as 2010, he walked with a cane, but he has since transformed himself into a downright beast. PD no longer slows him down. Since 2012, he's run over 100 half marathons, 15 marathons, and many other endurance races while raising more than $240,000 for Team Fox.[10] He's even taken part in *American Ninja Warrior*, a competition that only the very strong and fearless can even dream of entering.[11]

Though I couldn't help but feel like a lightweight next to these guys, I knew that it was the kind of company I should keep. We all had an affliction in common and the desire to do our part to help eradicate it from the world.

As I mentioned, charity runners are obligated to raise funds in exchange for their race entries. This is typically done by soliciting friends and family to contribute to the cause in the runner's name.

While sharing my 2021 WMM plan with some friends, I was encouraged to document the challenge in a blog. "It's the classic hero's journey," observed Howard. I don't deserve the "hero" label, but it was helpful feedback. The blog would be a useful medium for soliciting charitable contributions.[12]

Blogging about the adventure meant revealing my diagnosis to the world. Until my first post, I had told only family and a few close friends about having PD. Ultimately, I decided that it was useful information for others and so it was better to divulge than to keep it to myself.

In addition to soliciting funds, I intended to use the blog to update donors on my training and to recap each of the races. My posts started on July 2 and continued weekly until just after the New York City Marathon.

Like many aspects of this adventure, the blog surprised me. Though it served the purposes that I created it for, unexpectedly, some other treats came along. It was thrilling to learn that people were actually paying close mind to my exploits and eagerly awaiting then devouring my latest story within a few hours, often within minutes, of publication. Is this why writers write? It's energizing and empowering.

For me, writing my blog was one of the bonuses of this whole adventure. It didn't come for free, though. I felt an obligation to respect my admittedly small audience by writing with quality and, once the races began in the fall, by providing recaps in as close to real time as I could manage.

In return, my audience gifted me the act of reading my work, a gesture that I found to be nearly as therapeutic as running has been.

6

A Customized Training Plan

The training plan that I used for the 2019 CIM was a success. I followed it closely and hit the pace targets for each session as per the *Runner's World* pace calculator, and on my first marathon I came within five minutes of my finish time goal.

But my new goal was to run five of the World Marathon Majors in six weeks. This particular challenge is not covered in any *RW* training plan. Nor is the challenge of running the Chicago Marathon and the Boston Marathon on consecutive days.

Some modifications were in order.

Running back-to-back marathons is a thing nowadays and I found some compelling articles online describing how folks manage to pull this off. My research indicated that in order for me to run marathons on consecutive days then I'd have to run them slowly.

Yeah, ya think?

I thought there should also be an element of practicing longer distances on consecutive days. So instead of a single weekly long run I decided on doing two of them on consecutive days each week. For example, I started out with two 10-mile runs, one on Friday and the other on Saturday (10 + 10). The next week would be a 10-miler on Friday then a 15-miler on Saturday (10 + 15). For subsequent weeks I ramped it up—15 + 15, 20 + 10, 20 + 15, 20 + 20—and then tapered downward—15 + 15, 15 + 10, 10 + 10. I figured that if I survived the 20 + 20 week then I'd be in pretty good shape for Chicago and Boston.

Before all that, though, I still had some unfinished business to attend to.

I was registered for the 2021 Boston Marathon as a charity runner, but I still wanted to earn a bib for Boston based on my own merits. Why? Call it ego, midlife crisis, bucket list, or another chance to give a big FU to Parkinson's. Whatever. I like to set goals. I targeted Boston 2022 for that one.

The imbalance between the desire to enter Boston and the limited field size is a classic market demand situation and many marathons will actively promote their ability to BQ runners (i.e., their BQ%). For example, there are the BQ.2 Marathon Races in Geneva, Illinois and Grand Rapids, Michigan where odds are better than 50% that a runner will BQ. This is accomplished through scheduling the race for ideal weather conditions (i.e., 45-50 degrees with low humidity) and providing the logistical and fueling support that normally only elite runners receive.

Another compelling strategy is for the race to be run on a downhill course.[1] In 2019, of the top 12 marathons for BQ%, nine of them were on downhill courses. And four of these used the same course in the Cascade Mountains east of Seattle—the Palouse to Cascades Trail in Iron Horse State Park near North Bend, Washington. It's conveniently only a few hours' drive from my home in Seattle.

The trail drops in elevation gently and consistently just over 2,000 feet as it winds its way through the park. Most prominent of the events that use this course are the Tunnel Marathons of North Bend. These three races, held in June, August, and September, had BQ rates greater than 30%.

The effect of slope on a runner's pace has been quantified. Strava, the social network for recreational athletes, has done the big data thing on its users' records to relate a runner's mile pace on a flat course to her pace on a graded course (uphill or downhill). Strava calls it Grade Adjusted Pace (GAP) and reports it within a user's activity. A difficult uphill slog will have a faster GAP, which is the pace that the runner would have achieved running just as hard on a flat course.[2]

Flip the GAP data around to estimate the benefit of a downhill marathon. Using my own data, I've found that the -1.5% grade of the Tunnel Marathon course knocks about 13 seconds off my marathon mile pace. The first 2.6 miles of the Tunnel Marathon course is flat, so for the remaining 23.6 miles I'm likely to run a total of five or so minutes faster than on a level course—an enormous benefit toward achieving a BQ with some cutoff time margin.

But the benefit of running downhill comes at a cost.[3,4] Uncontrolled, that extra speed will generate more force on the body with each foot strike. And there is a tendency for runners to lean backward a touch to control speed. Because of the shift in the center of mass the runner now lands on her heels, which in turn causes the landing force to be absorbed in the knees and quads. It's a punishing way to run.

To compensate, the runner must bend forward at the ankles to match the torso's angle to the ground that it holds while running on a flat course. To protect his knees the runner must take shorter, faster steps. Without these corrections there will be serious muscle cramping and pain toward the end of the race and a correspondingly longer recovery period afterward.

I registered for the June 2021 edition of the Tunnel Marathon (aka "The Light at the End of the Tunnel Marathon"). And I also registered for the Super Marathon that uses roughly the same course to be held two weeks later. The latter race was a backup in the event of injury or cancellation. Originally, all I wanted was a shot at a robust BQ; I wasn't intending to run both.

But then I realized that doing two marathons two weeks apart would be a good way to start training for the WMM, which held events on consecutive weekends.

As it turned out they were two very different races.

⚬ ⚬ ⚬

Besides the downhill slope, the signature, and absolutely awesome, feature of the Tunnel Marathons is running through the Snoqualmie Tunnel. Formerly used for a railroad, it was abandoned in 1980 and is now part of a rail trail in Iron Horse State Park.

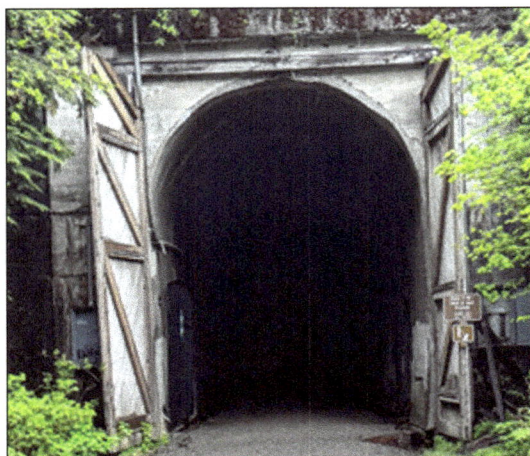

The Snoqualmie Tunnel (© J. Drake).

The tunnel is about 2.3 miles long and the course enters it early in the race. Whatever the conditions are outside, inside it's cold, damp, and very dark. Runners wear headlamps to see where they're going. But even with the headlamp it was difficult. I found that my breath would condense in a cloud in front of my face obscuring my sightline.

I experimented. Sometimes I held my breath to prevent the cloud formation, or I'd duck below or around my exhale to see past it. Mostly I just ran carefully while looking downward in front of me so that I might see and avoid ground hazards.

With at most 600 runners in these races the issue was not so much what was in front of you, as it was easy enough to avoid others. The real danger was underneath. At times, the ground was uneven, puddled, or riddled with potholes. One could easily trip or roll an ankle.

In fact, as I read online the day after, Arizona Senator Kyrsten Sinema broke her foot in the tunnel during a mishap in the first race.[5] I did see a runner hobbling after the tunnel exit but all I could offer her were condolences and a fist bump. Had I recognized her and not been in a hurry I might have taken the opportunity to speak with her about the evils of the filibuster.

The weather on that first run was ideal for me. Cool and rainy, I felt very comfortable throughout the race though I got thoroughly soaked. I slowed a bit near the end but I didn't really hit a wall. I turned in a 3:42:35.6, a BQ which could withstand up to a 7 minute 24 second (7:24) cutoff time. The cutoff time has never been as high as 7 minutes for the full Boston field. It was set at 7:47 for the 2021 race but that was mainly because the field size was reduced from 30,000 to 20,000 runners in the interest of pandemic safety. Field size should return to 30,000 in 2022 and with that, a reduction in cutoff time. This should do it.[6]

With my BQ in the bag, I was free to take it slow and easy on the subsequent Super Marathon. Tunnel aside, the course is stunningly beautiful replete with forest trails, waterfalls, and mountain vistas. I looked forward to taking it more thoughtfully this time around.

Good thing, too, for a couple of reasons. First, I woke up the day of the race with a back spasm. (I have chronic back issues that date to my late twenties.) Walking was painful and I considered withdrawing from the race. Ultimately, I decided to go for it anyway because, I don't know, what the hell.

Second, the Super Marathon was held on the weekend of the now infamous Pacific Northwest Heat Dome of June 2021. Race day temperatures were predicted at higher than 100 degrees. For safety, the director moved the race time earlier to 6:00 am in hopes of a cooler start and actively discouraged runners from seeking a BQ or a PR (personal record) that day.

That must have hurt considering that the BQ is the race's *raison d'être* but the director was keeping the welfare of the runners foremost. Additionally, more than the usual allotment of medical personnel was on the course this time in the event of heat-related injuries.

All in all, it was a good test of my plan to run at least some of the WMM at a slower pace than normal for me. Some friends and family suggested that I didn't have the wherewithal to rein myself in. They needn't have worried.

I found it easy to give myself a more leisurely pace. My fussy back helped me with that decision. At times I chatted with other runners, something I hardly ever do. And I stopped at each water station to drink several cups and walk a few hundred yards before picking up the pace again. Stopping is something I've never done on a race of any length, but it was more than appropriate this time given the heat and the BQ monkey already off my back.

I turned in a 4:23:37.6 for the Super Marathon, which would've been about 4:27:00 for a flat course like several of the WMM. Most of the WMM have a time limit for all runners at something like six hours. I'm good with that.

The heat took its toll on the Super Marathon field. The race website boasts a historical 34% BQ rate but this time around the unofficial tally was less than 12% (approximately 40 out of the 339 finishers). By contrast, with more ideal running weather, "The Light at the End of the Tunnel Marathon" two weeks before yielded 213 BQ's (40.5%).

So far so good. Two marathons in two weeks with no lasting ill effects. It was a start.

However, two long runs separated by two weeks is not at all like running marathons in Chicago and Boston on consecutive days. This doubleheader was the greatest physical challenge of the 2021 WMM and, therefore, the primary focus of my training plan. Rapid recovery was critical as was refilling the glycogen tank in less than 24 hours.

It was already clear to me that for rapid recovery, I had to run all the marathons at a slower pace than I normally would. I can do this. But how slow is slow? Slow is not an absolute. It depends on many variables, including the weather, how well I slept the night before, jet lag, etc.

I wear a Garmin Forerunner 245 watch when I run. It collects a lot of data that I review after each training session or race. I look for interesting and relevant patterns. My experience with the data suggested that with respect to rapid recovery, the most useful Garmin-collected parameter that I can use for real-time pacing is heartrate.

Like most runners, I can have bad days. I feel off during those workouts, my pace is disappointing, and afterward I'm sapped of energy and feel just generally crappy and useless for the rest of the day, if not longer. On my best days I feel fantastic. The run itself feels effortless and afterward I can be pleasantly helpful around the house.

I've noticed some correlations between my Garmin heartrate data and my good/bad days. First, I'm more likely to have a good day if I warm up carefully by running the first mile at a pace of 9.5 to 10 minutes per mile. I suppose that's partly why smart coaches urge their runners to warm up before any race.

Secondly, irrespective of warm-up, I've had bad days if my heartrate ever gets within 10 or so beats per minute (bpm) of my maximum heartrate, which I've determined through self-administered stress tests to be about 185 bpm. A good warm-up tends to prevent these heartrate spikes but not always.

For sure, I felt the need to steer well clear of my maximum heartrate in Chicago to have any chance of recovering in time for Boston. From examination of months of my heartrate data, I decided that rapid recovery from any race requires that I not allow my heartrate to exceed 150 bpm. I believe that this limit automatically adjusts my pace for the local weather conditions; that is, if it's a hot and humid day then I'll need to run even more slowly to keep the heartrate below 150 bpm.

I tested this plan on several of my back-to-back long run training days. On the first day I set my Garmin to alarm if my heartrate exceeds 150 bpm. When the alarm went off, I slowed down to allow it to drop below 150. This worked well on my 20 + 20 training week; there were no serious issues preventing me from running 20 miles on the second day. To more accurately represent the different terrains of Chicago and Boston, my first 20-miler that week was on a flat course and the second one was on a hilly course.

There are some fitness trackers on the market that use heartrate data along with skin temperature, respiration rate, and oxygenation to determine an athlete's readiness for exercise. The data is collected on a 24-hour basis, and much is inferred from data collected during sleep. Of considerable interest and utility is heart rate variability (HRV), a complex set of parameters that describe the many ways in which the heart is not strictly a metronome, and an analysis thereof can predict a body's readiness for exertion.[7] These trackers use HRV to, among other things, judge the adequacy of a night's sleep, foretell of an oncoming illness, and prescribe rest rather than exercise when the body is spent.

Could this data be of use to me with respect to Chicago and Boston?

No. Totally irrelevant in my situation. I already knew that by any rational metric come the morning of the Boston Marathon, my body won't be ready for another 26.2 miles. That's not the point; I'll be running regardless. The point is to prepare my body to have the best chance to finish the race. I believed that keeping my heartrate in check and fueling properly would give me that chance.

I practiced fueling on my 20 + 20 training week by carbo loading after the first 20-miler. Tissue repair was also important, so I ate protein in the magic 4:1 carb to protein ratio. I took copious notes. I believe that I ate 6,700 calories that day—a feat that rivals Thanksgiving. Sadly, it was not as pleasant a chore as I thought it might be. But it worked! I managed the 20 + 20 training week well enough.

Still, I had to plan out how to do this carbo loading while I hustle out of Chicago and fly back to Boston. I decided that I would eat the appropriate meal on my return flight to Boston. I would have to figure out how to bring that food onto the plane with me but that seemed manageable.

I have another, more personal, concern regarding "nutrition." If I'm out running for four hours, to stick to my medication schedule I'll need to take a few of my Parkinson's pills along the way. I've come to think of my PD meds as my performance enhancement drugs (PEDs) though not in the way that the United States Anti-Doping Agency (USADA) thinks of PEDs. Prescription medication use by recreational runners doesn't normally raise suspicions. I stash, oops . . . I store the pills in a small Ziplock bag that I carry in my clothing and use my watch alarm to remind me when to take them.

7

Clues

No one knows for sure what causes Parkinson's disease, though, generally speaking, it's believed that some cases are genetic in nature and others are due to exposure to environmental toxins.[1] I've often thought that my family is a great case study for the genetic version of the disease given that my father, myself, and two of my siblings have been diagnosed with it to date. I'm one of 12 siblings so it would seem the sample size is large enough to draw some meaningful conclusions.

There are several gene mutations that have been linked to PD with the most predominant being the LRRK2 and GBA variants.[2] I'm negative for those mutations as is at least one of my siblings who has PD. Most likely, then, we can rule out genetics as the cause of PD in my family. That's a relief to me because it means that my children are not likely to have it.

That leaves environmental exposure, but that conclusion does little to pinpoint a cause. There are many toxins that have been implicated and studied for their potential to cause PD: pesticides, heavy metals, chlorinated solvents, certain strains of bacteria in the gut, some neurotoxins,[3] and the list goes on. It's hard to unravel, especially because if there was any environmental exposure to our family in our household it likely happened decades ago, and any evidence is long gone.

I'm intrigued by PD research that implicates well water as a potential cause.[4] Growing up on Long Island, New York we had a private well. In the late 1990s, I saw a neurologist because of muscle twitching in my legs that I thought might be related to calf pain I was feeling. Discussions with the doctor inspired me to have our well water tested, which I did in 1999 and I still have the report from that test. We had coliform contamination as per the report, which means that there were bacteria in our domestic water supply but other than that no serious issues.[5]

There are many very smart people working the Parkinson's conundrum and I'm confident that they're making progress and will continue to do so until the cause and the cure are found. I'm hoping that eventually there will be an answer to the prevalence of PD in my generation of Drakes.

In the meantime, there are medications that a PD patient can take to improve their quality of life. As I mentioned previously, I take Sinemet, which is a combination of levodopa and carbidopa. Levodopa is processed by the body to make dopamine, the neurotransmitter that is in short supply with PD.

Once digested and circulating in the bloodstream, levodopa can pass through the blood-brain barrier (BBB) and enter the dopaminergic (DA) neurons where an amino acid, DOPA decarboxylase (DDC), converts it into dopamine.[6] Inside the DA neurons, this replacement dopamine is used by the brain's neural pathways to enhance the body's motor control systems.

However, neurons outside of the brain—in the peripheral nervous system (PNS)—also contain DDC and will convert levodopa to dopamine. Dopamine, however, is unable to cross the BBB.[7] Therefore, any dopamine in the PNS stays in the PNS.

Dopamine in the PNS is bad news. Unregulated by the brain, the dopamine in the PNS acts on neural pathways in such a way as to cause uncontrolled motions (dyskinesia) in the limbs of the patient. That's why carbidopa is combined with levodopa. Carbidopa blocks the action of DDC in the PNS so that the levodopa won't be converted until it gets to the brain.[8] The carbidopa is not 100% effective, however. Therefore, dyskinesia is a common side effect of Sinemet usage and worsens when the dosage is increased. The phenomenon is the basis of the myth that Sinemet's usage should be delayed as long as possible because prolonged use degrades its effectiveness. To be sure, Sinemet doesn't lose its effectiveness against PD over time. Rather, the increase in dosage required to combat the disease's progression exacerbates the side effect of dyskinesia.

I also take Eldepryl, the brand name for selegiline. Selegiline is a selective monoamine oxidase B (MAO-B) inhibitor. After use in the synapse, dopamine is taken up again by the neuron where it can be redeployed unless it encounters MAO-B, which degrades it thereby rendering it unusable. Inhibiting MAO-B prevents the degradation so that a single dopamine molecule will have longer term effectiveness.[9] When combined with Sinemet, because the available dopamine is reused, a patient can lower her Sinemet dosage thus reducing the risk and severity of dyskinesia. Thus, the patient's quality of life is often better when these two drugs are taken in tandem rather than through Sinemet alone.[10,11]

Most Parkinson's patients experience a return of their symptoms as the effect of the medications wear off. These "off" periods are unpredictable. Stress, anxiety, the timing and size of meals, physical activity, and other factors can all effect when and if an "off" period will occur.[12] It is such a common and disconcerting issue for patients that several new drug therapies have been introduced specifically to address it.[13,14] MAO-B inhibitors such as selegiline can help with "off" periods by extending the life of any Sinemet-derived dopamine.[15]

I have not experienced "off" periods since my diagnosis four years ago. I'm not sure why this is the case but it is possible that I am over-medicating. A personal dosage experiment is in my near future.

$$\sim\!\mathrm{CI\ \ I\!D}\!\sim$$

I don't present like a typical Parkinson's patient. Even before I started on medication, the tremor in my right arm was subtle and there were no other obvious external signs. Not apparent to others, though, were symptoms (e.g., muscle cramps, stiffness and stumbling when walking or running) that had been puzzling me for years.

I owe a lot to my siblings who were diagnosed with PD well before I was. Had I not become aware of their struggles, I may have inadvertently allowed a few more years of the disease's progression before seeking treatment.

Parkinson's disease attacks dopaminergic (DA) neurons in the substantia nigra (SN), a subregion of the human midbrain. It's been estimated that classic PD symptoms don't appear until 50% to 80% of them have died.[16,17] This may take the better part of a decade.[18]

Pre-diagnosis years can be frustrating. Peculiar changes arise for the patient that are hard to describe and, at least in my experience, create no resonance with a typical family doctor lacking the sufficient neuroscience background.

Starting in my early fifties, I had this weird thing going on with my left foot. Whenever I went for a run, at about a mile in my big toe would go into a cramp, locking up at a 90-degree angle bent at the knuckle. In another quarter mile or so the cramp would dissipate but until then running was painful and awkward. On some runs the cramp would return and, again, with a little more distance it would go away.

Naturally, I described this curiosity to sports medicine professionals but that went nowhere. The typical response was, "I've never heard of that." Well, they might have if they bothered to discuss it with a neurologist. It's called dystonia, it's one of many symptoms of PD, and it improved when I started on the meds.[19]

Dopamine also gets involved in many other functions, including behavior and mood. It's not unusual for PD patients to suffer from depression.[20] I did. I was treated with several different antidepressants and, for me, none of them were more effective than a nice, strong cup of black coffee. As I wasn't getting any useful help for the depression, I simply stopped seeing anyone about it.

I don't fault the medical community for a general lack of awareness of PD.

Or do I?

PD is not like heart disease, for example, a common and quantifiable ailment wherein there are tried and true objective diagnostic techniques and clear symptoms that even lay people are aware of. Early Parkinson's can be much more subtle.

Notwithstanding, I do think that physicians should get out more often. Maybe spend time with the specialists of other medical disciplines. I wonder how often an internist, as a random example, says to his patient something like, "Depression? Well, I can prescribe you some meds, but I think I'd like to send you to neurology. I want them to look into something for us."

Thinking across disciplines could make all the difference. Just like with heart disease, early detection of PD has the potential to improve a patient's quality of life. It would allow more people to get an early start on vigorous exercise, for example.

Within a few years of stepping up my exercise regime things had changed dramatically. Though my disease was never obvious to anyone pre- or post-diagnosis, I was beginning to doubt it myself. My symptoms were virtually nonexistent. My neurologist strongly recommended exercise as therapy but I didn't think that meant that I could make the disease vanish by running a lot.

It doesn't vanish; I still have PD. The neurons that died in my brain are still dead. I have PD symptoms though considerably diminished. I still feel dystonia in my toes although much less severe and without the debilitating cramp from my pre-diagnosis days. And there are times when I feel balance-compromised if I forget to take my meds on time. But my exercising may be extending the lives of my remaining DA neurons. It's become more widely understood within the medical field that this is the case—aerobic exercise can slow down and perhaps halt the progression of Parkinson's.[21]

It's long been medical dogma that the human brain undergoes development and structuring only during childhood. Relatively recent research, however, has shown that neuroplasticity (the ability of neural networks within the brain to change and reorganize) occurs in adults as well.[22]

John Pepper of South Africa had been having PD symptoms since 1963 when he was 29 though he wasn't diagnosed with the disease until 1992. In 1994, he began "fast walking" to the tune of about 15 miles per week. He credits his exercise routine for effectively quenching his symptoms such that he no longer needs medication.[23]

Pepper wrote a book, *Reverse Parkinson's Disease*, about his experiences with PD wherein he describes the regimen that has helped him, and others he has coached, to deal with the disease. He's not a physician, though, and his book and methods suffered the expected (possibly biased) fallout from the medical establishment.

Pepper's story is given scientific validation in *The Brain's Way of Healing* by Norman Doidge, MD.[24] There's much to unpack in this book but the claims are clear—the adult brain has the ability to protect neurons from degenerating and it can also strengthen and rewire existing neural pathways through an increase in certain chemicals brought on by enriched environmental stimuli (e.g., exercise, solving puzzles, creative expression, foreign travel, etc.).[25]

More recent studies support Pepper's observations.[26,27] Just Google "parkinson's and exercise" and millions of hits come up. I read one recent paper from researchers in the Netherlands who have found clues as to how the PD brain gets rewired via aerobic exercise and showed evidence of exercise's ability to reduce brain atrophy.[28] I emailed one of the authors to get some further insight. He believes that exercise doesn't resurrect any dopaminergic neurons but rather through exercise the brain makes better use of the dopamine that it has.

The apparent reduction in brain atrophy is an exciting area within Parkinson's research now. Exercise also stimulates the release of GDNF (glial derived neurotropic factor). GDNF is synthesized in the brain's glial cells, which are plentiful. GDNF has been shown to have a protective and restorative effect on the DA neurons in animal models.[29] Also, Vitamin D has been shown to increase the release rate of GDNF. My diagnosing neurologist prescribed Vitamin D3 for me and I've been taking 2,000 IU of it daily since then.

So, if its effects are truly restorative, why not just dump a bunch of GDNF into a Parkie's brain and cure the disease right there?

It's been tried and it hasn't worked yet. But there's still hope, and trials continue.

One possible reason for the current state of GDNF trials is the way in which it's been investigated to date. The research uses mouse models that develop a disease that looks a lot like PD when given MPTP, a neurotoxin that attacks DA neurons.[30] The GDNF helps to restore the dopaminergic neurons in these afflicted mice. But this is not how PD works in humans. Although neurotoxins can create PD in humans, not all PD cases manifest this way. And the sudden DA death in poisoned mice is unlike the slow degeneration of human Parkinson's.

There's a lot more to be learned here. This research highlights a serious difficulty with any kind of medical research. Testing on animals must occur before putting human patients at risk yet the results are not necessarily transferable.

In any event I believe that the copious running that I do is helping me live well despite having PD. Just like my diagnosing neurologist told me—exercise is great therapy. So, when it comes up, as it sometimes does, how I manage to run with PD, I have this explanation with its delicious circularity:

I run like I do despite having Parkinson's because I run like I do.

In fact, I would go as far as to claim that because vigorous exercise has been a mainstay for my whole life, my PD may have progressed more slowly pre-diagnosis than it would've had I been more inclined to the sedentary. In other words, it makes sense to me that a lifetime of exercise delayed the onset of my symptoms.

I need to be clear about one thing, though. It is not necessary for a Parkinson's patient to run marathons in order to reap the benefits of exercise. The current guidelines are much more modest. A regimen of about 120 minutes of aerobic exercise at 80% to 85% of maximum heartrate spread over three or four sessions per week has been shown to be effective at slowing the progression of the disease.[31,32]

There's another thing to throw into the mix. That same paper from the Netherlands researchers, and several other studies I've seen, suggests that aerobic exercise also increases reward-related activity in the brain.[33] Perhaps not too surprising given the role that dopamine plays in the brain's reward system and the popularized phenomenon of "runner's high." But you don't have to have PD to get that sensation.

8

The Killer App

Becoming a long-distance runner requires putting in untold miles over many hours, often lonely ones, to hone the craft. It's a challenge both in body and in mind. The mental aspect can be as overwhelming as the physical. Negative thoughts, such as fixating on the number of miles yet to go when the body is already complaining, will poison the effort.

It's a common issue for runners and I often wonder how I'm able to do it. To be sure, I don't entirely know. I'm new to this. However, I think that there are elements of deliberate directed thinking, a supportive environment, and a mysterious neurological effect involved.

It's important to stay positive, which I would argue is the crucial parameter that predicts success or failure.

The best marathoner in the world right now and perhaps the best there ever has been, Eliud Kipchoge, has the positivity thing dialed in. I've no idea what goes through his mind when he's outpacing the field, but I feel that there is a clue right there for everyone to see.

He smiles when he runs.

He has admitted that smiling is a trick he uses to coerce his body into pushing through the pain of a world class marathon effort.[1] The smile is an outward representation of a positive mindset, and the body follows along dutifully.

But what does the average runner think about that can summon a smile from the depths of discomfort? I don't know what Kipchoge uses but for me the thing that makes the most sense is love.

Love is mighty. It can do extraordinary things.

There are stories of ordinary people in times of extreme stress performing acts of enormous strength.[2] One thing that these acts have in common is love. Many, oddly enough, also involve automobiles. Love gives parents/children/friends the strength to rescue their children/parents/friends by lifting cars off of them.

When it gets rough, I think of what I love. My family. My friends. The breathtaking views I get when running around West Seattle. The fact that I'm retired and every day is a vacation. *The Killers*. Peet's coffee. A clever turn of phrase that I'll post on my blog. The trove of Garmin data I'll review at the end of the run. The nap I'll take after reviewing the data. The list goes on; there is no shortage of such things.

And here's the environmental observation that helps me keep a positive perspective. It happens every time I run a marathon, especially a large one involving thousands of runners.

I like to take in the scene. People, many of them, line the course. Except in very rare cases, they don't know me, and I don't know them. But they are cheering for me and my fellow runners nonetheless, clapping, shouting words of encouragement, and holding up handwritten signs that say things like "Smile if you peed just a little." And if any of us puts our name on our shirt or race bib those words of support come personalized.

It's kindness freely given by strangers who want nothing more than for everyone to do their best. It's empowering. And when you smile and wave back at them the kindness effect multiplies.

But there's no need to wait for race day to practice kindness. I've found that a friendly smile and a wave always works. Many runners I come across on training runs appear to have this figured out also.

So, I do my best to keep to this mantra: *Be kind and choose love.*

The mysterious neurological effect is, well, mysterious.

I've often admired the patience of artists, musicians, software programmers, and the like. For them, hours upon hours of concentration are necessary to create a beautiful and useful result. I've never had the patience for that though I've tried. My mind always wanders to other things that need my attention. To be in flow, that state of mind of being totally engrossed in a single task to the point of losing track of time and forsaking all other potential distractions has always eluded me.

However, as a marathoner, I'm somehow beginning to understand what flow is like. I focus on the task of running and lose track of time and before long, the run is over.

I've mentioned how exercise is great therapy for Parkinson's disease. My exercise regime, focused on running, has slowed the disease's progression in me and causes my brain to release more dopamine than it's able to do otherwise. The phenomenon has become widely known. There's a growing body of knowledge pointing to the benefits of exercise for all aspects of the brain, including cell growth, memory, mood, focus, attention span, etc.[3] Reward circuits are activated; that is, the brain finds the act of running rewarding.

From what I've learned on the subject, it seems likely to me that my brain uses the running I do to help me keep a positive attitude about the running I do. There's that circularity thing again. Like a perpetual motion machine, this phenomenon has the potential, at least I hope, to be inexhaustible.

It's occurred to me that if not for Parkinson's disease, I might never have become aware of how resourceful my brain can be.

9
The Pandemic Gauntlet

It was never a slam dunk that the 2021 Majors would even take place. Throughout the summer leading up to Berlin I read through news reports online to keep track of how the world was dealing with COVID-19. Particularly interesting were charts of daily infection rates as surge after surge swept through the world. Terms that all of us never before had to care about—herd immunity, virus variants, anti-vaxxers, green/amber/red country lists, and so on—were everywhere and around the world countries used these terms to develop and justify their new pandemic travel policies and protocols.

First to react with decisiveness was Tokyo, which on June 17 banished nonresidents from their scheduled October 17 marathon.[1] Japan decided to hunker down, bar the doors, and wait it out despite what havoc it may cause to their economy. At the time, it was a frustrating, seemingly over-reactive response given that the decision was made so far in advance of the race schedule with no inclination toward hope for things to improve worldwide well before October. In hindsight, it may have been a good call. Japan managed to keep their COVID-19 caseload extremely low throughout 2021.

Nevertheless, I still had a lingering, implausible hope that Tokyo would reinstate nonresidents into the October race. Then on September 17, Tokyo canceled the October race outright and moved it to March 6, 2022, which was the planned date for the 2022 Tokyo Marathon. So, the 2021 marathon would be held in 2022 and there wouldn't be any 2022 Tokyo Marathon.[2] Fortuitous coincidence. I'd already accepted a deferral from my tour operator to the March 6 event so my goal of running all the 2021 WMM was back on track even though one of those races would actually be held in 2022. It was a reasonable outcome considering that my original plan had been to run all six of the Majors in a single year. Running them all in six weeks would have been fabulous but five months would still be historic.

Vaccines became available early in 2021 but rollout was supply-limited and slow. (Lynn and I were serving as caregivers to her mother and therefore were allowed early access; I got my second Moderna shot in February.) Eventually those who wanted vaccination got it. The vaccines proved effective and around June daily case rates were coming down in Europe and the US. Mask mandates were lifting, and the European Union (EU) was talking about opening for tourism albeit with some testing restrictions. It appeared that the world was turning the corner on the pandemic.

Then came the Delta variant and by early August mask mandates returned in the US along with renewed calls for the unvaccinated to get the jab. But the states most at risk (in the South and in the Midwest) were no more likely to heed this guidance than they were the first time around. Being in low-risk, high-vaccination-rate areas, the US races appeared fairly secure albeit with the chance, as usual with my country these days, of things going sideways rapidly.

Germany as part of the EU and the UK, no longer so entwined thanks to Brexit, diverged in travel policy. In early August, Germany required mandatory testing for entry regardless of vaccination status, but by the end of the month vaccination had become mandatory at least for the runners in my tour group. The Centers for Disease Control and Prevention (CDC) advised against travel to the UK but didn't prohibit it, and despite much higher case rates there from the Delta variant, the UK wasn't placing any restrictions on vaccinated travelers.

As the time to board the flight to Germany was approaching, the whole situation was looking dicey and potentially risky for catching COVID-19. Until then, Lynn and I were planning to go to Europe together but in early September we decided that it wasn't worth risking it for both of us. Thus, the European leg of this adventure turned into a solo excursion for me.

In September, all the races were hedging their bets and stating publicly that they reserved the right to require face masks during the race. That's a pain but manageable. It's hard enough to breathe as is, but if it meant the races could proceed then I was OK with that. It was becoming clear that the US races weren't at risk for US citizens. Full vaccination would be required but they're going to go on with some health and safety restrictions.

Europe was another story, and that story was getting regular revisions.

In a nonbinding statement, the EU recommended that all member states ban nonessential travel from the US given its unabated rise in COVID-19 cases.[3] Germany didn't immediately respond with a ban. Yet, I was concerned that I might have to quarantine upon arrival. I considered the possibility of flying in two weeks early in order to have time to isolate before race day. The UK continued to operate unilaterally and there was no indication that any sort of ban was going to happen.

It was as if a continent-sized sphincter that controlled transit was poised over Europe and I needed to get through it, run Berlin, and get out before it pinched shut. Even if I did manage to achieve it, the passage was threatening to be unpleasant.

And then, heading into my departure date of September 22, all the lights turned green.

However, international travel was still complicated and volatile. There were many parameters and very few constants.

Destinations each concocted their own blends of science and politics to create "Red" (high COVID-19 risk), "Amber" (moderate risk), and "Green" (low risk) lists of countries thus describing the risks presented by arriving travelers. Toss in vaccination status, passport issuer, and itinerary for the previous 10 days to get the full matrix of travel restrictions a traveler had to contend with. Chaos!

Restrictions might include documentation of vaccination or COVID recovery status, COVID testing before arrival, COVID testing after arrival, quarantining, locator documents to facilitate contact tracing, online registrations, and what have you. It got confusing and more so because the situation was constantly changing.

In the end, despite a summer's worth of anxiety, getting into Germany turned out to be easy. I just registered on a German government website and then upon arrival I needed to flash my passport and CDC vaccination card and I was in. After Berlin, as I headed to London there would be a lot more COVID testing involved because the UK wasn't interested in vaccination status. I would need a negative PCR test before entry, another one within two days of arrival, and then some rapid tests to get into the race and the Expo. Then I'd need another PCR test to get back into the US.

There would be more of this at each of the race venues.

Universally, masks would be required indoors, on shuttle buses, and in the start and finish areas. And borrowing from music festivals (or maybe hospitals) many of the venues were adopting the practice of adorning runners with ID bracelets that signify that the participant had passed all COVID screening. These bracelets would be attached to the runner's wrist prior to race packet pickup. They'd guarantee access to the Expo and to the start area and were not to be removed until after the race.

Each race, though, had their own unique measures intended to reduce touch points.

Gear check got creative, wherein a runner could hand a bag of personal items (aka "kitbag" when in London) to a volunteer in the start area then collect it at the finish.

For loop-like races where the finish was near the start (Berlin and Chicago) gear check would be fairly traditional—on race day, drop off the gear before the start and pick it up at the end.

London eliminated the practice. Rather, each racer was required to drop off their kitbag at the Expo before race day. To help sanitize the familiar finish line rituals, race officials loaded swag, a race medal, and a T-shirt in each kitbag at the Expo. That would mean that the finish line tradition of volunteers adorning the necks of runners with medals wouldn't happen in London. Rather, the kitbag would be waiting for each runner to pick up, dive into, and create their own ceremonies with their medals and finisher shirts.

In New York City, the day before the race, a runner could drop off their gear near the finish line and retrieve it after running. Also, in a bid to avoid overcrowding, all runners were required to reserve a time slot for picking up their race packet at the Expo and for dropping off their gear that they'd collect at the finish.

In Boston, runners could check in their gear near the finish line before heading to the buses that would shuttle them to the start in Hopkinton.

None of these races (London, New York City, and Boston) would transport items, such as warm clothes worn pre-start, from the start area to the finish. If it was a cold day, runners could choose to either freeze at the start in their race attire or bring something warm to wear temporarily that they'd discard for charity before the start. This was new for London but traditional for New York City and Boston.

London had some other well-intentioned brainstorms. They advocated for runners to wear a commemorative belt to carry water with them while running thereby reducing touch points at the aid stations. The idea was that a runner could simply swap in a fresh bottle of mineral water at each stop rather than take a cup of water from a volunteer. London also proclaimed a highly unenforceable "one-supporter" policy whereby each runner designates a single person to cheer for them live along the course so that the streets wouldn't get overcrowded. I couldn't imagine any runner bothering to comply with this one.

In their official race instructions, the Boston Athletic Association explicitly requested that all runners refrain from kissing strangers at the halfway mark.[*] Uh, OK.

Still, it was all very exciting. Not only was I soon to get validation of my training strategy, it was also showtime for my logistics planning.

There were other issues, though. Even in normal times I have two personal concerns when travelling. The first is getting a good, nay, a great cup of coffee in the morning. If I'm going to Italy, not a problem. Italians know how to do espresso. But I can't feel good leaving this critical task in the hands of Germans (Berlin Marathon) or the English (London Marathon). Thus, I pack some Peet's and my AeroPress (a high-tech mash-up of a pour-over system and the traditional French press) when I travel to these countries. In fact, just to be safe, I'll bring my coffee and equipment whenever I'm on an overnight agenda anywhere.

The second has to do with the bed. My back has proven to be finicky ever since my late twenties when I first blew it out helping a friend move to a new apartment. Decades of periodic lapses into improper lifting of children, groceries, weights, etc. has left my back muscles recalcitrant. It's not unusual for me to wake up with an uncooperative spasm after spending the night on a hotel bed with its unfamiliar mattress. I couldn't afford that on this trip if I was to run these marathons.

---

[*] Providing this directive without any context was sheer, suggestive brilliance on the part of the BAA. Here is the missing backstory: Wellesley, a women's college situated close to midway along the Boston Marathon route, is renowned for its Scream Tunnel, where hundreds of students line the roadway to give a roaring emotional boost to the runners. This tradition has been going on, like, forever. Then sometime in the 2000s, some of the Wellesley women, in addition to cheering, began a new tradition of giving out kisses to the runners as well. Alas, the pandemic forced a cessation of this tantalizing courtesy.

In truth, the pandemic colored all travel plans with a broad brush of caution. Overseas excursions always involve keeping track of plane and train schedules, hotel reservations, and whatnot. In a new twist for 2021, I also had to keep on top of all the COVID testing required to allow my flitting about Europe, running the marathons, and returning to the US. I'm fine with this, though. Planning, logistics, and efficiency are my strengths. I'm big on developing a complex plan and executing it smoothly. However, given the stakes—the possibility of being denied entry into one or more races—there were anxious moments. Detailed planning is necessary but often it's luck that prevails.

Otherwise, I was set to go and looked forward to the mishmash of conveyances and the convoluted scheduling required to get me to the start lines on time with all the necessary paperwork, apparel, and equipment.

My personal highlight would be the doubleheader of the Chicago Marathon on October 10 followed by the Boston Marathon the next day.

By rule, all runners must pick up their packets at the Expo held prior to the race. Except for London, only in-person pick up by the runner is allowed—no substitutes. Specifically, I couldn't hang out in Chicago to prepare for that race while someone in Boston got my Boston packet for me. And I wouldn't be able to get back to Boston in time to hit the Boston Expo after running Chicago. The Boston Expo would be closed by the time I got back.

To be clear, I needed my Boston race packet in hand before I headed to Chicago.

My plan:

1. Fly to Boston on October 5 after the London Marathon and meet up with Lynn flying in from Seattle.

2. Continue my prerace training for Boston and Chicago while in Boston. Stay in an Airbnb Lynn found for us in a great spot, close to Copley Square and the finish line.

3. Pick up my Boston race packet with race bib at the Boston Expo when it first opens on Friday, October 8. Prepare my post-Chicago carbo-load meal(s).

4. Fly to Chicago solo (Lynn remains in Boston) on Saturday, October 9 and pick up my Chicago race packet at the Chicago Expo. Stay one night in the Hilton Chicago.

5. Run the Chicago Marathon on Sunday, October 10. Find a way to wash up afterward.

6. Fly back to Boston Sunday afternoon after the race arriving in Boston in the evening. Carbo load, hydrate, and nap on the plane. Stay in the same Boston Airbnb with Lynn as before.

7. Take the shuttle bus to the start line early Monday morning October 11 and run the Boston Marathon.

What could possibly go wrong?

I wasn't planning to set personal records (PRs) in any of these marathons because to do so would risk the goal of completing all of them.

Slow and steady finishes the race.

But I did have ambitions. Practically speaking, I needed to aim low for the Chicago–Boston doubleheader. These would be run at a pace that kept my heart rate below 150 bpm or something like 9:30 per mile.

It was tempting to aim a bit faster for Berlin because it was the first marathon, I wouldn't have beaten myself up yet, adrenaline would be running rampant, and the course is flat and fast. Similarly, I wanted to go for it in New York City because it was the last marathon. There was no reason to hold back. It seemed prudent to take London on the slow side so as not to jeopardize Chicago–Boston.

Hence, I set finish time goals of under 4 hours for Berlin and New York City and 4 hours 10 minutes for the others. The slower ones would still be nearly 30 minutes slower than my current PR of 3:42:36 set in June.

Truth be told, I would've been happy to come in anywhere near these times.

10

The Inscrutable Media

My digital news feed has picked up on the fact that I like articles about running and runners so I get a steady stream of them. They'll describe notable achievements by everyday runners, such as the earning of a sixth star, completing all the Majors in a single calendar year, running a string of marathons on consecutive days, etc. Irrespective of the PD angle, I'd a notion that my challenge ought to be of similar interest to other runners.

Ever since the compressed schedule for the 2021 Majors was set, I thought that there would be more runners who recognized the once in a lifetime (hopefully, once in forever) opportunity it represented and that I would have company in running all of them. But all through the summer of 2021 there were no reports of anyone taking on the challenge. I was beginning to think that my journey would be unique.

Thinking that it would help with my fundraising and my blog views, I sent out a few teaser emails to some publications, online and in print. I even mentioned it directly to some of the marathons when, for example, they surveyed participants for the inspirations that led them to run in their events.

Mostly, I got crickets.

If the lack of interest was due to skepticism, I could certainly understand that. Those who didn't know me could be forgiven for questioning my chances for success. Until the fall of 2021 I had run a total of three in-person marathons plus one virtual. The only indicator of my seriousness about the challenge came via publications to my blog that I started in July of that year. However, I don't have a large social media presence, each of my weekly posts were getting only a few hundred views, and most of them were from family and close friends. I wasn't on anyone's radar.

In mid-September, I got a nibble from the New York Road Runners (NYRR), the organizers of the New York City Marathon. Laura Paulus of NYRR Public Relations told me that my story impressed them and that they may like to source it to various media outlets. That process would heat up closer to the NYC Marathon date but in the meantime, Laura followed my progress through the rest of the events.

But then on the brink of the Berlin Marathon, the media suddenly got very interested in the 2021 WMM.[1,2,3]

On September 20, just six days before Berlin, Shalane Flanagan announced that she was going to run all the World Marathon Majors on the compressed schedule. Nike sponsored her and the challenge was dubbed Project Eclipse.

Shalane is a 16-time United States champion who, among her other accomplishments, won the New York City Marathon in 2017—the first American woman in 40 years to do so. She retired from professional racing in 2019, but apparently, she wasn't done with running.

To be clear, Shalane had taken on the same challenge that I had but with some notable twists. In place of running Tokyo, a race that was postponed to March 6, she would run a virtual marathon on October 17, the original Tokyo date, to make it six marathons in six weeks. She also announced that she planned to run each of the Majors in less than three hours. Evidently, she had started planning and training for this effort about the same time that I did early in the year.

My chagrin was two-fold. Although I had no problem with her finish time goals—I don't live in the sub three-hour world—I did think that the virtual marathon in place of Tokyo was gratuitous. Five marathons in six weeks seemed sufficient. Not to be outdone, I thought, what the hell, and signed up online to run the Seattle Virtual Marathon and put it on my schedule for October 17 also, six days after we were to complete our Chicago–Boston doubleheader.

What's one more marathon after all?

More exasperating than the self-imposed sixth marathon, however, was the media coverage that Shalane received. She got a lot of press, articles featuring her were showing up relentlessly in my digital news stream, and here I was wallowing in obscurity despite attempting essentially the same feat. The unfairness gnawed at me.

By then, I'd already embraced the idea and practice of maintaining a positive mindset. It helped me in my transformation into a long-distance runner, I've reason to believe it's excellent therapy for Parkinson's, and I'm happier. Positivity requires deliberate attention to my mental state. Nowadays, when I recognize darkness gaining advantage, I'm compelled to reverse it. For having grown up on Long Island, New York, the land where grudges go to find eternal life, this is no trivial task.

Love displaces hate. Charity over greed. Hope, not despair. Smiles, no frowns. I don't pretend that this works for everyone in all circumstances. But I feel better when I've successfully morphed a dark emotion into its positive counterpart. Does positive thinking slow down PD? Well—sure, let's go with that. Negative thought can't be therapeutic.

This new development tested my positivity. I struggled with it, and I could feel the resentment taking control of my mindset. Sometimes on my training runs I'd be so preoccupied by the whole situation that I couldn't concentrate on my workout plan. It was uncomfortable, unproductive, and untenable. I needed to get past it somehow.

So, I flipped it into admiration.

Actually, that was relatively easy to do. And a hell of a lot easier than dealing with resentment.

I knew as well as anyone how difficult it was to train for this challenge. But I'm retired and our kids are on their own. Other than my marriage I have no high priority demands on my time. Shalane is a full-time mom and a coach; kudos for taking on this challenge as well.

And, from what I read in her press interviews, the effort rekindled her love for the sport. Relieved of the pressure to reach the podium, she could enjoy the thrill of running for the fun of it. This could be exactly the inspiration that anyone who suffers burnout needs in order to renew the perspective that got them into running in the first place. It extends beyond running; it could be applied to any other profession or pastime for that matter.

Also, after her retirement in 2019, Shalane had both of her knees surgically reconstructed. Getting back to form meant a lot of work. Oh, and the three-hour finish time target? Only in my dreams would I be capable of that no matter how hard I trained on my relatively unscathed knees.

There was plenty to admire about Shalane's challenge. On top of that, she'd done me a favor—having the same goal as a goddess of American running validated my own. Besides, Shalane's presence in my story makes it a far more interesting tale than it would be without her.

Cool. Pity-party over and the real party was about to begin. Off to Berlin and the start of the adventure.

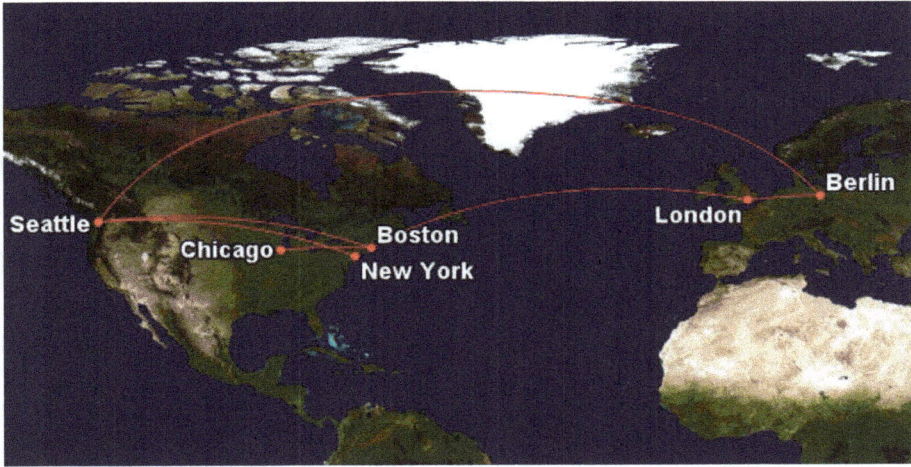

The Flight Plan for traveling to all the World Marathon Majors: Seattle to Berlin to London to Boston to Chicago to Boston to Seattle to New York City to Seattle (© J. Drake).

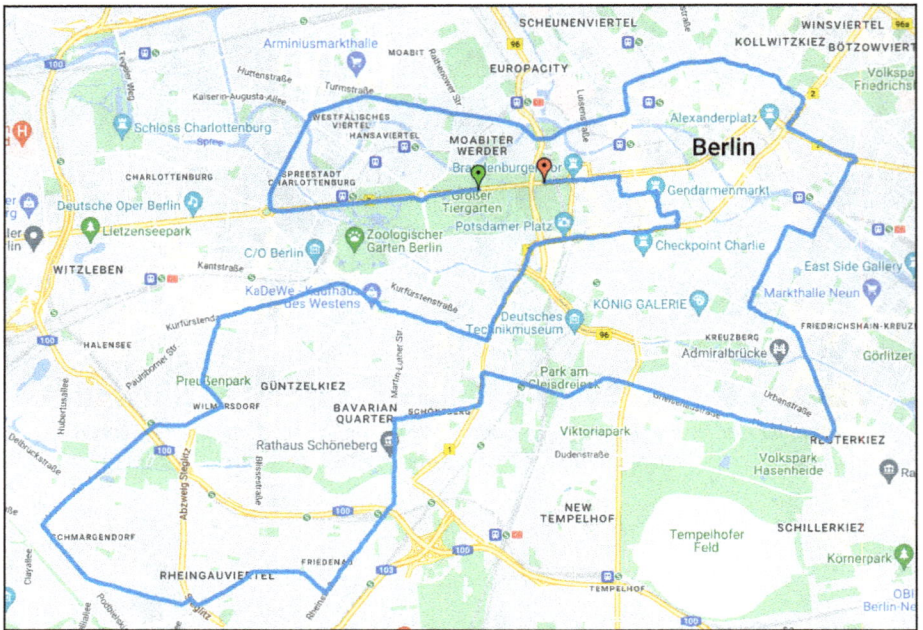

The 2021 Berlin Marathon Route (© J. Drake).

11

Berlin

A little beyond the halfway mark of the Berlin Marathon the temperature had already risen at least 10 degrees from what it was at the start. My heartrate had spiked well above my comfort zone, and I needed to make some adjustments.

At the time I was guzzling water at one of the many stations on the route and got the idea to douse myself to help lower my core temperature. The water was cold on my head and neck but felt comforting after the initial shock.

Another runner decided to get in on the fun, so she tossed her cup of water at my chest. That first time was cute and a little funny until she went back to the table to get some more water. Giggling the whole time, she must have dumped four cups on me.

The cold shock to my chest made speech impossible but I managed to gasp out enough of a message to get her to disengage.

This water table escapade may have been the high point of the race for me.

Marathon Tours and Travel (MTT) is the International Tour Operator that I worked with to gain entry into the Berlin Marathon. The President, Jeff Adams, and Trip Designer, Nicole Langone, had the mind-bending job of navigating the volatile currents of the pandemic while keeping these tours on track.

MTT arranged a reception on the Thursday evening prior to Sunday's race. I was expecting a small, intimate group of runners on this tour. I don't know why I thought that. I must not have been paying attention. In fact, there were about 100 runners among us and nearly as many who came along to support them.

I'm a committed introvert. That doesn't mean I'm shy or antisocial; those are misnomers. Introverts tend toward quiet introspection and are more likely to listen than to speak. Still, being alone is no bother. We thrive in pandemic-enforced lockdowns, for example. This evening I anticipated grabbing some food, listening to the program-related announcements, then heading back to my room to read email.

In the right company, though, my inner conversationalist shines. In one of the first of several unexpected bonuses of this whole adventure, I found out that much to my delight, marathoners are wonderful company.

Having not been a marathoner until recently, I had never before been amongst such a large group of them in a social setting. I shouldn't stereotype based on this one tour group, yet it struck me that recreational marathoners had to be the friendliest, most supportive people I could ever hope to meet. Everyone was kind, eager to chat, and interested in each other's stories. It helped that we all were fluent in the language of running. One runner I met, Suzanne Barron,[1] likened the experience to an adult summer camp.

Dumb luck may be at work putting me in such situations but it's up to me to do with them as I will. I decided that I was going to make the effort, during the entire adventure, to be uncharacteristically talkative and approachable. I'd smile and initiate conversation with anyone I came across. There seemed to be little risk, everyone was so kind, and the upside was clear—this was an amazing, and potentially enriching, opportunity to meet extraordinary people from around the world.

As expected, there were others who had divined the opportunity in the compressed schedule for the Majors. Many runners I met were planning on running more than one of them during these six weeks. Each had their own plan as to how to recover in time for their next race. Very few who were running multiple marathons were very concerned about their finish times.

I was amazed at how many runners suffer the Imposter Syndrome—the feeling of somehow not being deserved of a title despite abundant supporting evidence. Rosie O'Sullivan is the perfect example. In her lovely Irish lilt (she now lives in Connecticut) she says, "Oh, I don't think of myself as a runner." And then she proceeds to tell me how, at the age of 79, she's run 114 marathons (Berlin will be 115), including all 50 states and five of the seven continents.[2]

I shared my story with Rosie and that turned out to be a nice way to contribute to the conversation. I did the same at the reception where I met Karyn Ryan and her husband, Mark. Karyn is the runner and Mark came along to support her. They took particular interest in my challenge and asked for a link to my blog, as did Suzanne earlier. Somehow Karyn manages to train for marathons despite the five children that she and Mark are forever shuttling about town.

Most of the folks were travel weary so the reception didn't last all that long. I went off to bed ecstatic and grateful, that in a short time, some of the runners I met contributed to my Team Fox campaign.

The next day (Friday) held more opportunities for socializing: breakfast, a tour of Berlin, and the visit to the marathon Expo to retrieve our race packets.

The hotel served a traditional German breakfast buffet, enormous, with such a diversity of foods (e.g., pastries, breads, fruits, cheeses, eggs, meats, etc.) that anyone's ideal of proper fueling—as long as it wasn't dependent on well-brewed coffee—could be easily satisfied. I suppose that's not fair of me; I didn't taste the coffee. I just knew better.

I struck up a conversation with John Porter, his wife, Carol, and Steven Howard, all of whom were lawyers and longtime members of a running club in Houston named PRx. They'd run several of the Majors and had some welcome advice for me. For example, waiting at the start in New York City will be cold so dress warmly. Also, bring along a $20 bill with you in New York so that afterward you can buy one of those great soft pretzels that are sold from carts on the street.

Both John and Carol were tentative about Sunday's race because they were nursing leg injuries. No matter, they were enjoying themselves even if it turned out that they'd have to scratch.

The Berlin tour took place immediately after breakfast and ended with the stop at the Expo. Most of the folks on the tour still seemed to be dealing with some jet lag. I'd made my coffee in my hotel room in the morning, so I was all set but Suzanne and another runner, Stephen Evans, were getting desperate for an espresso and snuck off at one point for a fix.

The tour took in a lot of sights that we'd run by on Sunday. The marathon course winds its way throughout all of Berlin, a city iconic for its roles in World War

II and the Cold War. But in place of the "death strip" where, prior to the fall of the Berlin Wall, East German citizens were gunned down by soldiers on watchtowers if they attempted to cross into West Berlin, there now are fabulous new structures steeped in symbolism.

Here are some examples:

- The German government is housed in the Chancellery. It's the largest government building in the world and a wing of it bridges the river that formerly separated East Berlin from West Berlin.

- The Reichstag, which contains the Bundestag, the lower house of Germany's parliament, has a glass domed roof and a citizen's open viewing balcony directly above where the political machinations take place. The arrangement is intended to suggest government transparency.

- The Holocaust Memorial is a mesmerizing cartesian array of 2,711 concrete slabs of differing heights covering 10,000 square meters. From a distance, the slabs all appear roughly the same height but the ground they rest on slopes downward, so wandering into the memorial the slabs appear to grow in height eventually dwarfing the visitor. The effect is one of a gradual but ultimately overwhelming ascendancy much like Nazism, a metaphor proposed by our tour guide that feels apt.

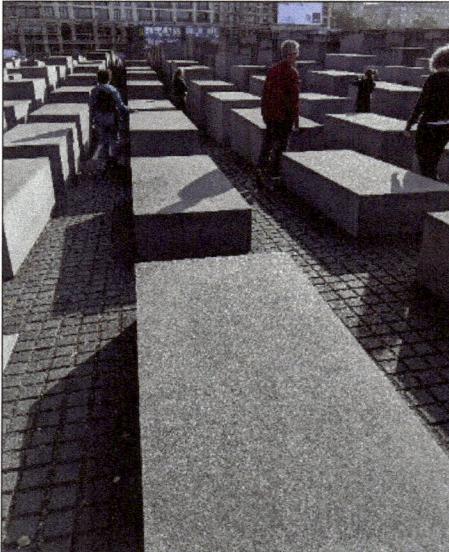

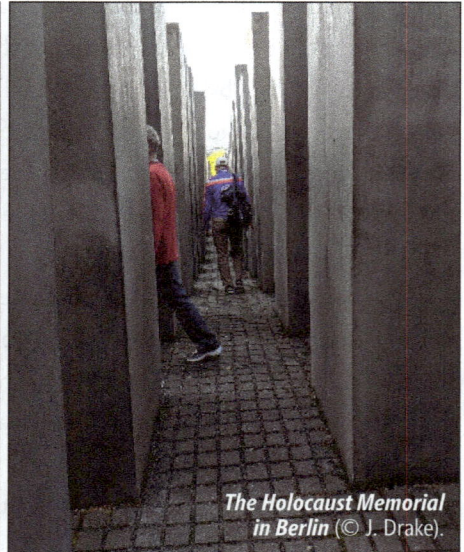

The Holocaust Memorial in Berlin (© J. Drake).

- Nearby the memorial is the site of Hitler's bunker where he spent his last days. It's a scruffy, unpaved, and unmarked parking lot.

During the tour we came across an enormous crowd protesting for action on climate change ahead of Germany's general election that weekend. Greta Thunberg was on hand to give a speech at the Reichstag.[3] I didn't know that Greta would be in Berlin at this time, but I sure did feel relieved and smug about my decision to buy those carbon offsets back in February.

Our trip to the Expo revealed a process incongruous with the expectation of German efficiency. It was my first on-hand exposure to how these huge events were dealing with the need for pandemic safety. Entry to the Expo required first a paperwork check (i.e., identification, vaccination, or COVID test status) and then the adornment of a wristband that allowed free access to the Expo and the race thereafter. Race officials opted for a serial processing model for these two steps with very little parallelism so there was a long line for the paperwork check followed by another long line for the wristband. This was for entry into a building that was still about a quarter mile walk from the building that housed the Expo. Once in the Expo there was another lineup to receive our race packets.

Was this really the best that Germans could do?

Also, in a curious and cumbersome policy, Berlin runners are required to carry a timing chip secured by laces to one of their shoes. These are "rented" for the race and runners are to return them afterward. If you forget to return them (as I did) you are fined the purchase price of the chip. For those of us who knew only of the free radio-frequency identification (RFID) emitter affixed to the backside of our race bibs, this felt like opportunistic larceny.

Suzanne and I were running in London the following week so we both opted to take a PCR COVID test at the Expo that we could use to get us into the UK. And, once again, another long line. I expected a different approach in Germany, one with higher throughput. But it wasn't a serious problem, really. Everyone was pleasant and helpful so the time passed without stress.

The Expo itself was fun although, we were told, downsized relative to pre-pandemic Expos. HOKA was there and though it was a week before the release of their new Bondi X shoe, a marriage of their flagship Bondi product and a carbon fiber plate, they displayed and sold them proudly. I ran around the Expo in a sample pair. Not enough of a trial to know if they're the real deal but no red flags, and I'm eager to add them to my pile of training shoes.

~⬡ ⬡~

As is typical of prerace training, I went for a couple of short runs on the days leading up to the event. I ran in the Tiergarten, a public garden about the size of New York's Central Park where the marathon's start and finish would be, which was not far from the hotel. It's a great place for a run with many paths and features (e.g., statues, sculptures, ponds) to provide variety. I had a little bit of back pain from the hotel bed but I felt OK running. Disturbing though was my unusually high and spiky heartrate for such easy, slow runs. It wasn't due to heat because I ran in the morning before sunrise. Perhaps my body was feeling jet-lagged. I don't know. I shrugged it off at the time because there wasn't much I could do about it other than run slower if my heartrate got too high.

The evening before the race, MTT hosted a dinner for more meet and greet and a chance to top off the carbs. My new friends from Houston invited me to join them at their table so I got to know them a bit better. Theirs seemed a fun club to be part of. Besides John, Carol, and Steven there were James and Brooke Williamson, who had come to Berlin with their toddler son, Cooper, and Brooke's mom, Jan Sizer, who came along to help out. John and Carol were still tentative about the race but were going to make the final decision in the morning.

I liked their strategy of bringing a young child to Europe with them. Lynn and I also made a point of traveling with our children, Kinsey and Aidan, when they were very young. That helped them to become confident and savvy international travelers as adults.

Brooke is a lawyer also and started running with PRx when she was a student about 10 years earlier. James is the odd non-lawyer in the PRx crowd that I met. He works as an insurance underwriter for Ascot, a Lloyd's of London Syndicate. There may have been some kind of tacit protectiveness for Brooke amongst the other club members. To hear John tell it, Brooke had a lot of PRx aunts and uncles watching out for her when she and James started dating.

At the dinner there was talk of cloud cover at race time so that temperatures wouldn't get too bad. In fact, it was quite comfortable as James, Brooke, John, and I walked to the starting line, maybe mid-50s (Carol had decided to scratch). But by race time it was heating up with no clouds in sight. It would eventually get into the mid-70s.

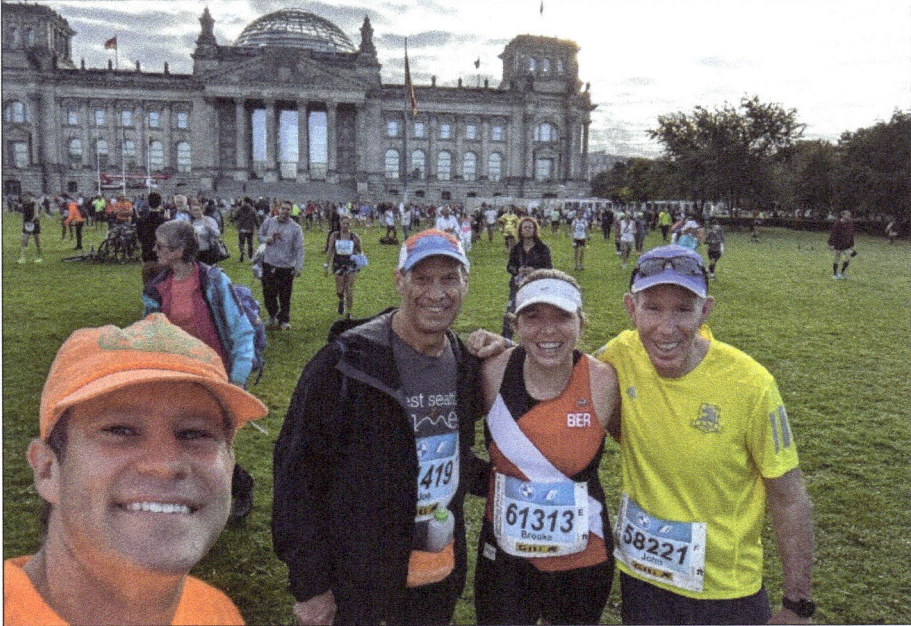

James Williamson, Joe, Brooke Sizer Williamson, and John Porter in front of the Reichstag just before the start of the 2021 Berlin Marathon (© J. Williamson).

Heat didn't seem to trouble the Houston folks. For them, mid-70s is like the mid-50s for someone who trains in Seattle—lovely. I don't do so well in the heat, and I know that I gain misplaced confidence from running well in the coolness of the Pacific Northwest. But as decided earlier, my plan for these races was to let my heartrate be the metric for pace and I would maintain it below 150 bpm.

I had understood that runners were forbidden to use hydration packs during the race. That was true for the other Majors, but it wasn't until the day before the race that I read that Berlin allowed them.

How did I miss that?

Could have made a big difference but, alas, I left mine stateside. However, the experience was undoubtedly more entertaining as a result.

Berlin promoted itself as the first large scale marathon to return in the COVID-19 age while obeying the constraints placed on it by the virus. Our wristbands secured our entry to the starting area, but we were asked to wear face masks at the start and again at the finish.

It was indeed a massive scale. Twenty-five thousand runners and, it seemed, nearly as many volunteers managing it, highly efficient gear check procedures, and untold thousands of portable toilets. Like with the gear check, the expected German efficiency (at last!) was on display with their toilet strategy. Open-air urinals were set up alongside the more private unisex portable stalls to allow the less modest men to do their business quickly thereby decreasing overall queue time for all facilities. Pretty neat but unlikely to fly in the more prudish UK or USA.

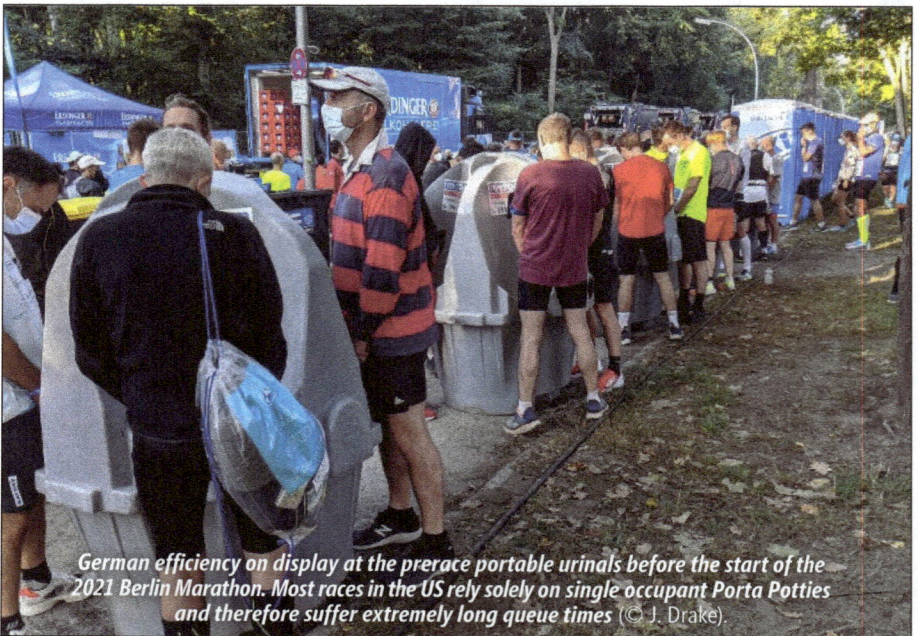

German efficiency on display at the prerace portable urinals before the start of the 2021 Berlin Marathon. Most races in the US rely solely on single occupant Porta Potties and therefore suffer extremely long queue times (© J. Drake).

The show was apparently broadcast to all of Germany. Huge Jumbotrons were set up and we could watch the crowd of us waiting for our turn and check the status of the lead runners who had already been sent off. At one point while waiting for the starting signal, shoulder-to-shoulder with other masked runners, I was nudged aside politely but insistently as a roving camera crew sought to interview an attractive young woman standing next to me. I assume that they had no interest in attempting an interview with me because somehow they realized that I didn't speak German. Yes, that must have been it.

During the race, the spectators were outstanding. They lined the entire course and cheered nonstop. Various bands played, people sang and danced. Some in the crowd made the effort to read the name on bibs and shout personalized encouragement. (Berlin was the only one of the Majors that had the runner's first name printed on the bib in a size large enough for spectators to read.)

Sometimes it seemed, the exhortations went a little darkly. James felt that the locals were particularly harsh on any German runners who decided to walk a bit and called them out by name for it. Apparently, James surmised, that was expected of the non-Germans but not so of the countrymen.

Normally, I'd have some Nuun electrolyte tablets dissolved in my hydration pack water that I could leisurely enjoy during the course of a long run to ward off leg cramps. I did bring some tablets with me and a small flask to fill with water from the aid stations on the route. The tablets were too big to fit through the flask opening and I lost one of them trying to break it in half so it would fit. In any event, I didn't bring enough tablets for the race because I was expecting I'd have some electrolyte-based drinks at the water stations.

Not so. My bad, I didn't read the race information closely enough. There was something besides water at the refreshment stations, something tea-like but unknown to me. Sticking to the marathoner's creed of "nothing new on race day" I chose not to risk possible GI tract distress.

The leg cramps came on about halfway in and steadily increased in severity through the rest of the run. My pace dropped off as my walk-to-run ratio drifted upward. By the last two kilometers, after passing through the Brandenburg Gate with the finish line in sight, I felt like I was barely moving.

And then I wasn't at all. At least not forward. With 50 meters to go my legs seized up and I hit the ground while the crowd's cheering gave way to a collective gasp.

I made up that last part about the gasp, but you get the idea.

Several runners came to my aid and helped me up but standing was very difficult; the muscle cramps took control of my legs. It appeared as if the other runners were going to help me across the finish line, but I put an end to that. With the end so close, I was going to finish that race on my own steam.

I stumbled across the line while my helpers stood nearby. Some First Aid folks were waiting for me and asked if I wanted to go to the Medical Tent. I tried to brush them off, but my walking was slow going and the course officials were getting anxious about me clogging up the finish area.

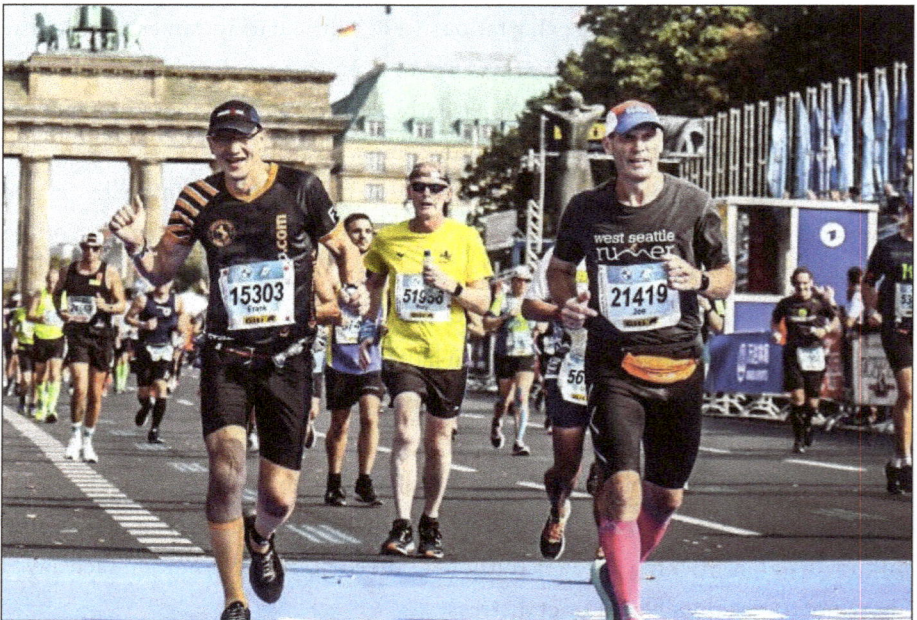

Closing in on the finish line at the 2021 Berlin Marathon (runner #21419). This photo was taken just seconds before I fell due to leg cramps that had become horrific over the last 10 miles (© J. Drake).

This is how I came to experience the inside of a marathon Medical Tent. The people there were very nice and helpful although, true to form, they'd no electrolytes to offer. Well, they did have a sports drink to bring me but what I really needed was something with fewer carbs that wouldn't upset my stomach. Like some of my favored Nuun tablets. Or a salt lick. They monitored me with concerned expressions as I lay on a cot while my legs were ravaged for about 90 minutes with the most severe cramps that I could remember.

I chatted with John Pasdois, a French IT expert in CyberSecurity, on the adjacent cot who also had some trouble with the heat though he was able to leave the tent well before I was ready. We exchanged contact information and I was thrilled to see his texts come in after every one of the races asking me how they went. Great people, these runners.

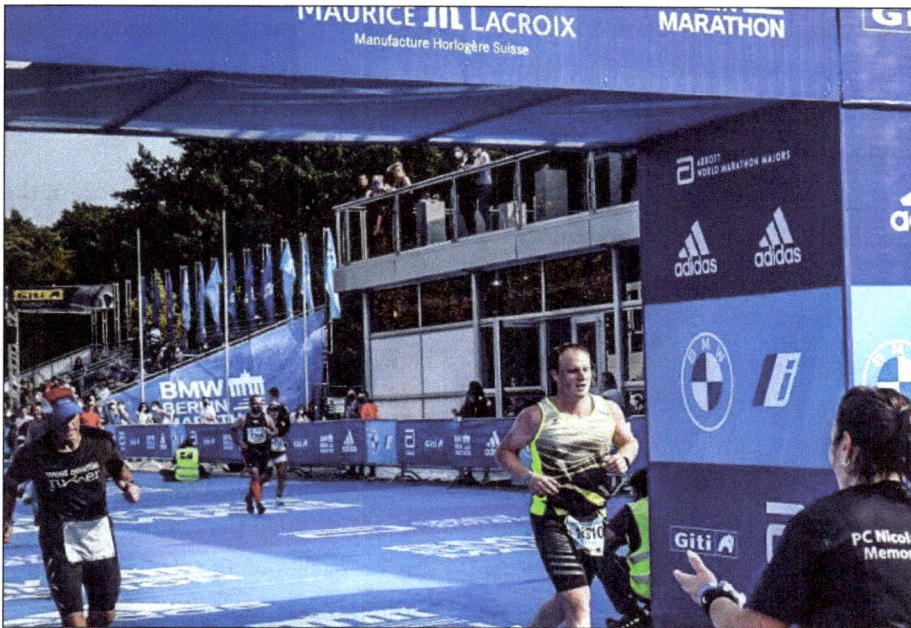

Crossing the finish line in Berlin (I'm to the far left). Some things to note in this picture include the lady in black cheering for me. She is one of the runners who helped me to my feet after I fell. Regrettably, I didn't get her name. And look at my bib that has fallen, and my number is no longer visible. Normally, race photos are matched to runner using the bib number. But in Berlin they did the matching using facial recognition software (I sent them a selfie of my face). Without using AI, retrieving this photo would have been impossible (© J. Drake).

Someone mentioned the race medal, which I hadn't yet picked up because of my detour to the tent. That motivated me to get moving (cramps be damned!), pick up the medal, reclaim my gear check bag, and amble back to the hotel.

To be sure, evidence of the toll the heat had taken on the participants abounded. Medics were assisting runners on both sides of the finish line and some runners were being placed on stretchers. Normal, I suppose, for an event of this size.

The tour's postrace party was in full swing by the time I returned to the hotel and showered. Feeling drained, nauseated, and light-headed I still wanted to see how the other's had done; I'd be leaving for London early in the morning, so this was my last chance to touch base.

Brooke, James, Suzanne, Rosie, Steven, Stephen, and Karyn all came through fine. John's leg let him down, so he eventually scratched but was unperturbed. I tried to eat a bit and have a beer, but my nausea quashed that. We all swapped stories of the races and I told of my finish line debacle and the incident at the water station. Carol had a better water station story from a previous race where some nasty runner pushed her aside to get water for himself and the volunteer stationed there threw a cupful at his face justifying her action afterward by saying, "He looked hot."

I found out that another runner in our group had also fallen just short of the finish line. He too got up and finished the race on his own power.

The marathon created an app for supporters to use in tracking their favorite runners, and friends and family used it to check my status throughout the race. I was and I am still touched by their dedication because stateside, regardless of which coast they were on, they had to be up during wee hours to keep tabs on my effort. Some European friends encouraged me by text real time. But many were following from abroad and I found out later that they became anxious as my pace slowed during the latter miles. From this input, I decided that in the upcoming races I would post a selfie from the finish line on Facebook in real time so that I don't worry them unnecessarily should something appear amiss.

What else did I learn from this run?

Well, given my finish line difficulties perhaps there was some more evidence that what I was attempting was insane. Even more so if London went the same way. I had a week to figure out what I did wrong and fix it.

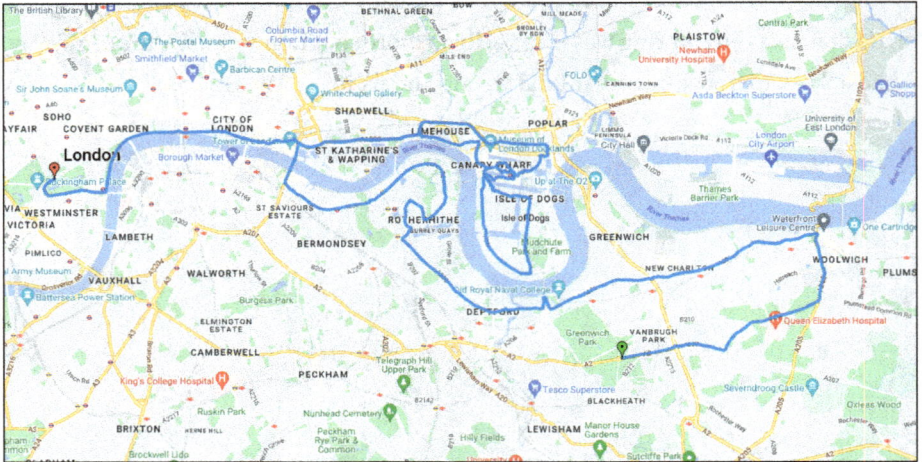

The 2021 London Marathon Route (© J. Drake).

12

London

The day after Berlin was busy. The results of the PCR COVID test that I took at the Expo came back negative, so I was free to enter the UK. I had scheduled my flight for 6:55 am (why did I think *that* was a good idea?), well before the hotel's ample breakfast spread was available, hence I missed that treat and settled for the coffee I made in my room. In truth, it didn't matter much because my stomach was not yet ready for a meal.

Queueing at check-in I fell into conversation with a German diplomat who'd been working relations with England for more than two decades. Very entertaining in an unsettling way. Currently it was all about the consequences of Brexit. That week there was a big trucking mess at British ports. Imports were being held up on arrival to the UK because there was no oil coming in to fuel the trucks to haul the goods away. Besides that nightmare, the gentleman had the pleasure of working on the Iran nuclear treaty under Obama and the dismantling thereof under Trump. He was looking forward to his retirement coming up.

Once in London I made my way to my Airbnb, prepared to wait it out until check-in time at 3:00 pm. I finally felt well enough to eat so I grabbed one of those strange English breakfasts that included a side of beans. Weird, yes, but it was my first real meal since Sunday's marathon, so I tucked in. By the time I finished I found out that Lynn had arranged for early check-in for me so off I went.

At that time, travel rules to the UK called for getting a PCR COVID test within two days of arrival. An accepted approach was to have a PCR kit sent to the traveler's UK address, obtain the DNA sample, then mail it to a lab for analysis. I ordered the kit while in Berlin but, somehow, I got the wrong address for the Airbnb and though I tried mightily to get it corrected, the testing company sent it to that incorrect address two days before I arrived in the UK. No doubt it was lost, and I was thinking I would need to get another kit but there was no guarantee I'd get it within the prescribed two-day window.

I decided to try my luck. And why not? My planning attempt didn't work this time. Perhaps luck would prevail.

I found the London address where the kit was sent. It was an apartment unit with one of those intercom systems for allowing entry. Buzzing some unsuspecting occupant didn't seem wise, so I just waited outside for an opportunity to pounce on the open door once a tenant exited. My chance came within 15 minutes. As a gentleman came out of the building, I held the door open while I explained my situation. Unruffled, he checked his own mailbox and a parcel with my name on it was there. My test kit! Luck, it seems, did prevail. He handed it over to me without further ado.

I'm almost certain that I could have ignored this particular test requirement with no repercussions. The system seemed sloppy enough that my noncompliance would surely not be noticed. Fortunately, I didn't have to test that theory. It was a relief to get that sample prepared and mailed off so I could turn my attention toward more food and rest.

I closed out the long day by writing and posting my recap of Berlin to my blog. It was published more than a day after the end of the race, so I felt a bit neglectful of my supporters. However, considering that for my stateside friends it was just midday the day after the race, I felt that they'd give me a pass this time.

In the morning I was better able to appreciate my surroundings. Lynn booked me a great Airbnb in SoHo close to Hyde, Green, and St. James Parks therefore I had some very nice scenery for my training runs. It was also close to the finish line near Buckingham Palace, which would make the walk home after the race uncomplicated.

While resting after my morning recovery run in St. James Park, I thought about what might have gone so wrong in Berlin. Sure, it was hot and that led to dehydration and cramps so that's understood. But I've run in conditions like that before and I've never felt so miserable as a result. What really happened? I knew that the temperature was high, so I monitored my heartrate and whenever it went over 150 bpm I slowed down, and to compensate for the heat I drank a lot of water at every aid station and . . . oh, right. Duh! Electrolytes. How did I miss that? This had become a frustratingly frequent question during my journey.

As the body sweats, sodium must be consumed to replace the sodium lost in the sweat. This is done to maintain the electrolyte balance across the cell membrane.

What happens when there's not enough sodium in the fluids surrounding the cells?

Well, then there's an electrolyte imbalance with a higher concentration inside the cells than outside of them. As a result, water is absorbed by the cells, and they swell up putting pressure on the surrounding tissues.

What about, hypothetically, when it's a hot day during a marathon and the runner drinks a lot of water, and I mean *a lot* of water, without completely replenishing the sodium?

That spells trouble. It leads to a condition called hyponatremia where the body's cells expand so much from water buildup that the pressure on the surrounding tissue can cause some very serious problems. The brain is particularly at risk—a sudden pressure buildup in the brain can lead to encephalopathy, which can cause death.[1]

Hyponatremia is also known as overhydration or water poisoning. Symptoms include muscle cramping, nausea, vomiting, fatigue, weakness, headache, confusion[2]— your basic shit show.

This is something that I'd known already from a theoretical point of view. I can't explain why it didn't come to mind during the race. I'm happy to report that I'm now intimately aware of the symptoms in practice thanks to my poorly conceived and sloppily executed hydration strategy during the Berlin Marathon.

It was an embarrassing newbie mistake.

Turns out, I'm not alone. While in London I read a study done on a random sampling of runners of the 2002 Boston Marathon and 13% of them had hyponatremia during the race, some of them severely, and this skewed heavily toward newbies with finish times greater than four hours who drank a lot of water during the race.[3] I'm sheepishly raising my hand here.

Elites don't typically encounter this issue because they have the experience to know better and they have trainers to reprimand them when they do something foolish.

The good news is that the risk can be completely avoided with a well-considered hydration plan, which I didn't pay enough attention to in Berlin.

I scolded myself for the oversight. For the 2019 California International Marathon, I'd studied up carefully. I reviewed all the information provided by the race website and had my fueling planned and executed down to the milligram of sodium and gram of carbohydrates. What happened to my world class sense of anal retentiveness? Certainly, if I was planning on trusting the on-course fueling stations then I should've been explicitly aware of what products they were serving and how I would use them. Inexcusable. More entertaining for future retellings of the tale perhaps, but still, inexcusable.

I decided that it really was about time to start taking this 2021 WMM challenge seriously.

At the hotel's fitness room in Berlin, I had access to foam rollers but not so at the Airbnb in London and I really needed one. The roller is a nice alternative to a massage for helping the leg muscles recover. I tracked down a running store and bought one along with a bunch more Nuun tablets for hydration and some Maurten 100 Gels. I decided not to trust any in-race nutrition in London. I'd carry everything I needed except for water.

My plan this time around was to stop to refuel roughly every three miles at a water station. I'd carry a 300 ml flask in my Flipbelt (a tubelike carrier made from a stretchy fabric that is worn around the waist) filled with water from the station and a Nuun tablet. The tablet needs a few minutes to dissolve, and I didn't want to wait for that so after drinking up I'd add another tablet to the flask along with a splash of water so that the tablet would be dissolved and ready for the next pit stop. I knew from Berlin that the tablet is a larger diameter than the opening on the flask, so the day before I would split the tablets in half so they'd fit easily.

At each stop I would down a Maurten 100 Gel to provide the carbs needed for the latter miles of the race. As appropriate, I would also take any PD medication that was due at the time.

I practiced the strategy on my training runs and it worked fairly well. I carried the flask with the dissolving Nuun in my Flipbelt positioned at my lower back. When dissolving in water the Nuun tablets fizzed off some CO_2, so if the flask was sealed tightly the pressure would build inside and the flask would expand putting uncomfortable pressure on my lower back. Therefore, I learned to leave the flask's lid open just a crack to allow the gas to escape. Some of the sticky, concentrated Nuun water would also escape so that was a little messy but not too bad. All told I could count on losing two to three minutes at each pit stop but that seemed a worthwhile price to pay to avoid a Berlin sequel.

These lost minutes made me wistful for the support that the elites get when they run these races. They're just handed their preplanned nutrition to gulp down in stride.

The next order of business was to unravel the COVID testing requirements for the race. I needed to get a lateral flow test to enter the Expo. Unlike Berlin, London chose not to go with tamper-proof wristbands to absolve the runner of any further testing, so I would need another one to enter the starting area. The test was self-administered and self-reported. Results were ready in one hour and had a 48-hour shelf life. Therefore, one strategy was to take the test on Friday and apply it to both the Expo and the race. But I'd a lot of stuff going on Friday, so I planned to do the test on Tuesday and pick up my race packet at the Expo Wednesday and retest later in the week for the race.

But it wasn't clear where to obtain these tests. The marathon website didn't make that clear and a Google search gave all sorts of cumbersome, pricy options though my understanding was that the test was free. I discovered that libraries dispensed the kits but the two I visited were fresh out.

The librarians sent me to Boot's, which is akin to CVS or Rite-Aid in the US. All the Boot's pharmacies in London gave out, for free, boxes that held seven test kits. Problem solved. Interesting system, though. The test result is reported to the UK's National Health Service (NHS) for tracking purposes. Each test kit has a unique QR code stamped on it; reporting is done by scanning the QR code while on the NHS website and indicating whether the test was positive or negative. But there were no checks against submitting false results. A runner in the London marathon might not even bother to perform the test and simply scan the code and declare it negative. No one would be the wiser.

It was a curious reliance on the honor system to control the spread of COVID-19—an approach that has been shown repeatedly to be flawed during the course of the pandemic. (For the record, I returned to my local Boot's on Saturday for the PCR test required for me to return to the US after the race.)

I tested an honest negative on COVID-19 and got to the Expo on Wednesday where London's logistics exceeded expectations. Whereas Berlin single-streamed the obtaining of race packets and bibs resulting in bottlenecks, London relied on massive parallel processing and therefore lickety-split thru-times. It helped make up for the cumbersome COVID testing protocols.

Like Berlin, the London Expo was downsized compared to prior years. A nice feature in London that Berlin didn't have was an hourly stage presentation on the Expo floor where speakers presented a slide show to familiarize runners with the race morning's activities. It answered a lot of questions and left at least one unsettled. One slide showed a very long queue to a portable toilet and the speaker stated that this one was atypically short.

"If you see a line this long," he urged, "get on it."

Helpful advice, surely. But why were the London Marathon organizers so accepting and, apparently, given that they made no attempt to conceal it, prideful of this obvious inconvenience? No point in debating the issue, though. It was unlikely that the speaker had any influence on the situation. I resolved to arrive to the starting area early.

With my race packet obtained I now had plenty of time to dive into the fantastic array of cultural opportunities that London presents. Time, yes, but not the energy. My body had not yet recovered from Berlin. Consequently, the rest of the day Wednesday and most of Thursday were rather quiet. I did, however, spend some time in both the British Museum and the National Gallery. And I got some appreciation for the various London neighborhoods while walking about. I now know why Warren Zevon has werewolves walk the streets of SoHo in search of Chinese restaurants.[4] The SoHo district includes both London's Chinatown and my Airbnb; SoHo is *the* place to get a big dish of beef chow mein.

On Friday I was very busy tramping around the city for meetings. First off was a morning chat with Vitor Rodrigues, a friend of a friend of ours from Palo Alto.

A software engineer at Google, Vitor is also a cheetah; he was shooting for a sub 2:30 PR in the race. Besides London, he had a few races lined up stateside in the following months. He was binging on running in advance of a planned hiatus after the birth of twins due in February. After the race he texted me that he'd spent some time running alongside Shalane Flanagan and noted that she had a sizable support crew with her. He was impressed that I was handling all the logistics myself.

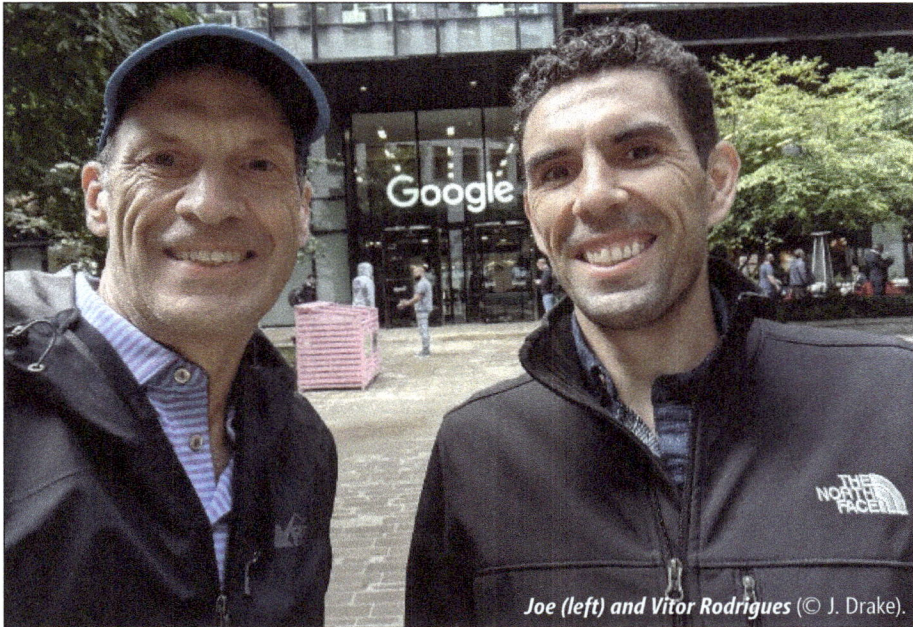

Joe (left) and Vitor Rodrigues (© J. Drake).

Pardon the digression but an anecdote here seems appropriate. It may help to illustrate something about my nature.

A few years ago, I drove with Lynn to a niece's wedding and upon pulling up to the venue I spotted a sign indicating that parking was to be performed by valet. I muttered something to the effect that I didn't need anyone to park my car for me as I dropped Lynn off and drove to the lot. When I returned on foot Lynn was chuckling with some of the other Drake wives. They were all terribly amused by the fact that all the Drake brothers, upon reading that sign about valet parking, responded exactly as I had and parked their cars themselves.

Implicit independence, often stubborn and sometimes clueless, is in the Drake DNA. Or at least in our Y chromosomes. I suppose that if Nike or some other deep-pocketed benefactor had offered to assist me with my World Marathon Majors journey I may have considered it. The fact of the matter is that it never occurred to me to ask for help. Why would it?

Self-reliance is double-edged. It can do serious damage to the uninformed or unprepared. Reluctance to ask for sorely needed help has led to many a downfall.

Yet, one shouldn't presume too much. Requiring assistance is like seeking permission. It suggests a limitation that may not, in fact, exist.

How does one learn one's limits if not for testing them with solo exploits?

At the age of 58, in my marathon debut, I coached and trained myself to a BQ finish. I will be forever insufferably smug about this achievement. The task may have been easier and more decisive had I employed a coach; however, I don't think it could possibly have been more satisfying.

For the 2021 WMM, I received support in many unforeseen ways. These were gifts that I welcomed and will always cherish; however, I may never have experienced such love without, first and foremost, a steadfast and clueless disregard of my limitations.

After leaving Vitor at Google's London offices, I headed off for lunch with some of the Team Fox London runners (Michael Blum, Melissa Loh, and Natan Edelsburg) and our leader Liz Diemer,* Team Fox Director. Liz is very good at her job. Cheerful, friendly, smart, and energetic, she juggled her schedule to create several opportunities for Team Fox members in London to connect before the marathon. Michael, Liz, and I came to lunch on our own but Melissa and Natan both brought their young kids, while Natan's wife, Caroline Hershey, also joined us.

I managed to get backstories on the other Team Fox runners. Natan is the Chief Revenue Officer of Muck Rack, a high-tech company building tools for public relations professionals to interact with journalists. He's a big fan of Michael J. Fox, is passionate about marathon running, and his wife's (Caroline) grandmother had PD so Team Fox was a natural fit for him. Natan ran in Berlin the week before, and also planned to run New York City in November.

---

* Liz has since been promoted, well-deservedly, to Vice President.

Michael Blum is an attorney with Stanley Black & Decker and got hooked up with Team Fox through his friend, Bret Parker, who I mentioned earlier (see Chapter 5, Team Fox). Besides London, Michael had run for Team Fox twice before in New York City.

Melissa lives in Maryland and is a former lab researcher and high school chemistry teacher, now a stay-at-home mom. From her father's side, an aunt and an uncle were both diagnosed with PD. Her aunt has passed but her uncle lives in Taiwan and with COVID travel restrictions she has been unable to help him. Running for Team Fox gives her desire to assist the Parkinson's community an outlet.

Team Fox London would meet again for drinks in Leicester Square that evening but, in the meantime, I had a Zoom call with Team Fox Boston. I took the call in a coffee shop (I ordered safely: hot chocolate). This would be my only chance to meet the team before Boston's race because I needed to be in Chicago while the prerace meetup was happening. Another great group of people—Aaron Parker, Max Shinsheimer,[5] Eric Gesimondo, and Alexis Maharam (who missed the call, but I'd meet her by chance later)—as well as our organizers from MJFF, Liz Berger, Melanie Barrett, and Katie Casamassina.

It was Aaron's wife, Bethany, who had the dream of running for Team Fox in Boston given that her dad, Steve, was diagnosed with PD in 2016. She would have done it in 2020 but the pandemic killed that effort and, in the meantime, she developed adventitial cystic disease that limited blood flow to her calf. An artery bypass surgery initially solved that problem but it was only a temporary fix and it has kept her from running. So, in steps Aaron to continue the fundraising effort and to take her place on the course on race day.

Eric's story is particularly inspiring. His father, Jesse, owned a hair salon and day spa services business in Natick, which is at mile 11 along the Boston Marathon route. Jesse had started with very little and built that business, Jesamondo Salon & Spa, into an extended family of over 40 hair stylists and spa professionals. Twenty years ago, Jesse was diagnosed with PD and Eric watched it take his father from him over the course of those two decades. Jesse passed away the previous April. In honor of his dad, Eric ran for Team Fox in Boston and proudly witnessed Jesse's legacy as he came upon mile 11 amidst signs, cheers, and the screaming roar of "Jesse's girls."

When Michael, Liz, and I regrouped for drinks, I met the stars of the show in London: Bill Bucklew (US) and John McPhee (UK) who on the following day would complete their epic collaboration *The Long Walk for Parkinson's*, a 670-mile trek over the course of 17 days that started in the northern reaches of Scotland and ended in London. They did this to raise awareness of PD and $100,000 for Parkinson's research. Bill capped this effort by running in the London marathon the day after finishing the trek. Bill and John both have PD. They were great company. We enjoyed a pint while a camera crew circulated around us capturing the stars of *The Long Walk* at rest.

Over some Guinness, the discussion turned to a topic I've pondered a lot recently: What is it about Parkinson's that inspires so many of us to attempt such physically demanding feats? Dopamine lust no doubt is one explanation. It's easy to get hooked on euphoria. And there's the growing realization that intense physical activity can slow the progression of the disease. Bill, who was diagnosed nine years ago at the age of 43, remarked to me that his doctor is amazed at how slowly the disease has advanced in him.

The physical exploits suggest that these Parkies aren't in their right mind, an apt description of the affliction if there ever was one. Maybe the damage to the substantia nigra imparts just enough crazy into the Parkie's mind that these enterprises are met with cheerful anticipation and stubborn determination.

Could it be, however, that this phenomenon is more fundamental and universal to human nature than merely a feature of Parkinson's?

Parkinson's places into focus our mortality not unlike cancer, multiple sclerosis, or any other incurable disorder would. Given a clearer view of the rapidly approaching horizon, I know that I've heard an insistent voice in my head saying, "Dude, what are you waiting for?"

That voice has compelled me to say "Yes" to challenges and exploits that I would have dismissed offhand before my diagnosis. And after a successful execution, and the corresponding hit of dopamine, my instinct is to raise the bar. Surely, I'm not the only one who feels this way.

It just so happens that when these challenges involve vigorous exercise, PD is held at bay. What's not to like?

I must interject here: The trend set in Berlin of meeting the kindest, most supportive people one could hope for continued unabated in London. In a way it's not too surprising given that those I met are into marathoning and either work for or are running for a charity that they're passionate about. But it's still unexpected and delightful. On top of that, everyone was extremely positive toward, inspired by, and I dare say, in awe of, the challenge I was working through. These really are great people.

I think all of Friday's walking put a latent toll on my as yet unrecovered body. On Saturday morning my back was a little stiff and then I did something extremely stupid. The Airbnb's bed frame shed some slats, so I attempted to lift out the (heavy) mattress to repair them and that did it. My back went into a painful spasm. Beds can always find a way to get to me. With the race the next morning this was very much not good news. I did some stretching and some foam rolling in an attempt to loosen up my back with little effect.

I knew from experience that spending the day in bed hoping that my back would heal was a futile strategy. Often, movement is the better therapy. Thus, I went off to meet *The Long Walk* crowd in Hoxton Square as we planned the evening

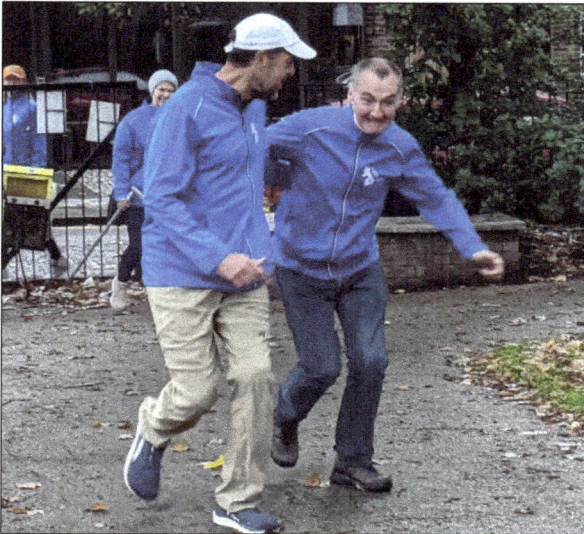

Bill Bucklew (left) and John McPhee (right)
finishing their Long Walk *for Parkinson's (© J. Drake).*

before. All my new pals from the previous evening were there along with a BBC TV crew sent to document the completion of the campaign. But standing around was tough going for me so I slipped away quietly and headed home to do what I could to rest and repair my back before my next appointment.

Dinner was with another Team Fox runner, Jeremiah Mushen, and his wife, Anne Marie. Jeremiah thoughtfully made us a reservation at a Chinese restaurant in SoHo right around the corner from my Airbnb thereby saving me some time and wear and tear on my back.

Jeremiah and Anne Marie live in Seattle; Jeremiah and I touched base earlier in the summer. He was running in honor of his uncle, Bill, who battled Parkinson's for 25 years up until his death. Jeremiah is extremely fast and was invited to run in the Age Group World Marathon Championships being held coincident with the London Marathon. I imagine he could've run in London without needing a charity bib, as he seems fast enough, but he's really committed to the cause.

We had dinner on the early side given our race in the morning. The starting line for the marathon was out in Greenwich, which was a train ride away from SoHo. In a gesture that the other World Marathon Majors cities should adopt, a runner's race bib allowed free transit on London trains all day.

My back was still in a snit when I woke. I have mentioned before that putting on knee-high compression socks even in the best of times can be a challenge. Finger strength and mechanical leverage are required. However, a back spasm trebles the challenge. When my back is like this, it's hard to bend at the waist and just getting into a position that allows me to reach my feet becomes a painful and comical enterprise. My strategy is to sit on the floor with my back against a wall while slowly, gently reaching for my foot with a sock in my hand. It takes a minute or so for the muscles in my back and legs to stretch to the point that I can touch my toes. Once there, in what seems like an eternity filled with pain, gasps, and grunts, I'm able to force the sock over my foot and up to my knee. From there I'll rest a bit before working on the other foot.

All the more reason to get an early start on the day.

My train to Greenwich left from Charing Cross, which was a short ride from the tube station at Leicester Square. Walking to the tube was slow and disconcerting. If

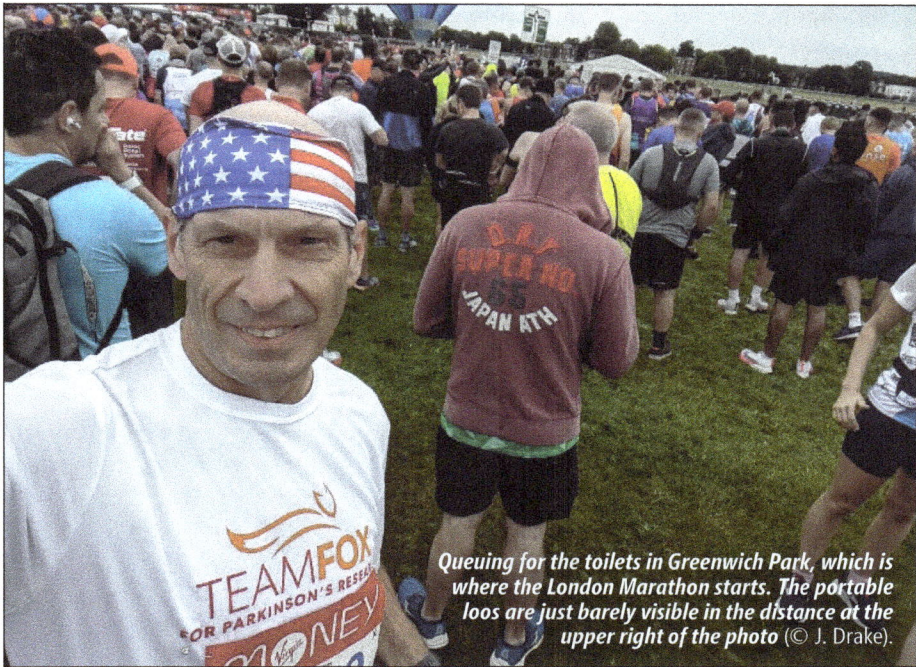

Queuing for the toilets in Greenwich Park, which is where the London Marathon starts. The portable loos are just barely visible in the distance at the upper right of the photo (© J. Drake).

my back didn't start cooperating soon, the marathon itself would be ghastly. While on the train, however, and chatting with a race volunteer, the spasm miraculously dissipated. Brilliant! The volunteer's job, by the way, was to act as a "sweeper." As sweeper, her unenviable task was to end the race for entrants who were unable to meet London's seven-hour cutoff time for finishing.

As advertised, the lineups for the portable toilets in the starting area were ridiculously long. Queue time was at least 30 minutes. It's not uncommon for nerves to prompt a second trip but by then I did stumble upon a latrine area, remote and rather hidden, with the kind of male facilities akin to what Berlin used. A more prominent advertising of the latrines could've saved many runners considerable waiting time.

The race atmosphere in London was remarkably similar to Berlin's. Thousands of spectators lined the streets to cheer on the runners, the crowd-limiting "one supporter" policy notwithstanding. Bands played, drummers drummed, people sang. It's impossible to overstate how helpful the spectators are. It's like running through a forest of joy.

London, however, had more costumed runners than Berlin. I saw a rhinoceros, a giraffe, a pair of scissors, several buildings, a unicorn, and the list goes on. At one point I passed The Flash and felt rather smug about that until he pointed out that he'd already completed the course once and was on his second lap.

Team Fox set up a cheer station along the route led by Liz. The folks at the station cheered crazily when they saw one of the Team Fox runners come by. But the crowd of runners was thick, and it was hard to spot individuals. I should've tried harder to be noticeable, as I was barely visible, but that didn't stop Liz and I from screaming at each other as I ran by.

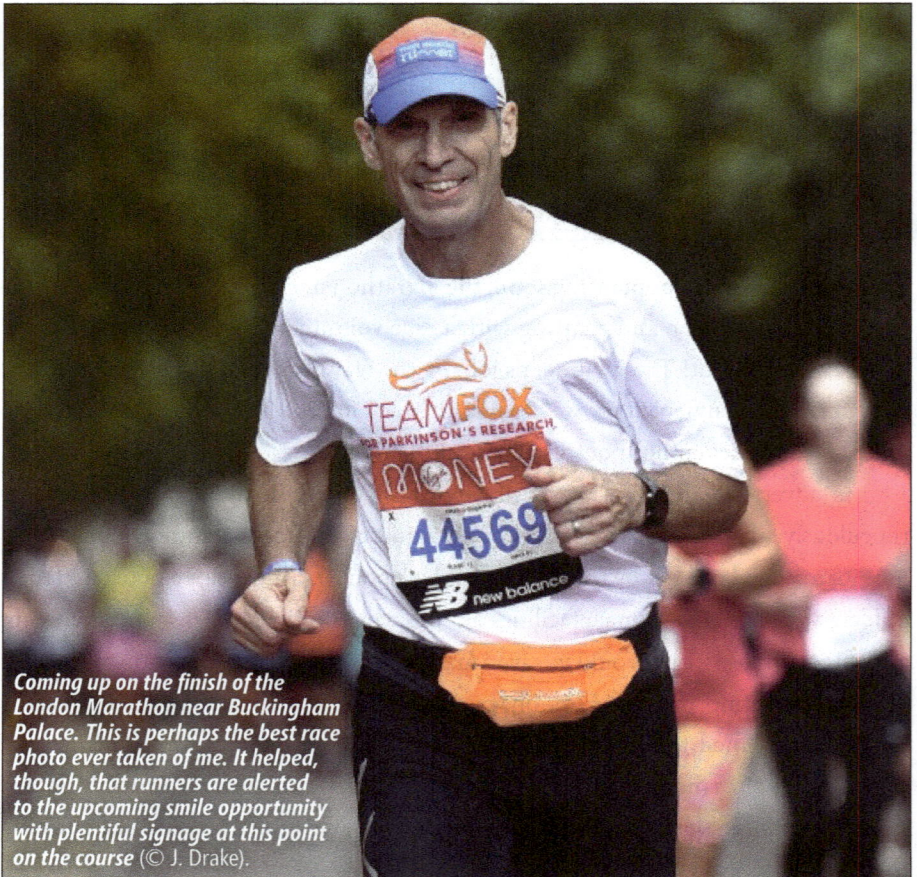

Coming up on the finish of the London Marathon near Buckingham Palace. This is perhaps the best race photo ever taken of me. It helped, though, that runners are alerted to the upcoming smile opportunity with plentiful signage at this point on the course (© J. Drake).

This time my hydration/nutrition strategy worked well so there was no repeat of the week before. The cooler temperature (52 degrees) undoubtedly had an impact. I shaved off about 18 minutes from my finish time of the earlier race and the leg cramps that so possessed me in Berlin were exorcised. Also, my pace throughout held fairly constant so the wall that I hit in the last few miles wasn't so sturdy. A light, refreshing rain fell for the last mile or so leading up to the finish near Buckingham Palace. Though sore, my legs were much better off at the finish than they were in Berlin.

Afterward, I crashed the postrace party at the Strand Palace Hotel for Parkinson's UK, MJFF's local partner. It was close to the finish line, and I really wanted the shower and the hot meal that they offered. I hadn't planned for this, however, so I had no clean clothes to change into after the shower except for the race's finisher's shirt that they'd stashed in my kitbag at the Expo. At the buffet, though, my shirt and I fit right in, and no one seemed to mind the sweaty shorts and socks I wore. My postrace nausea wasn't as bad as it was in Berlin, so I forced down some food knowing I wasn't going to be up for foraging later.

Melissa was there also so I got to see her children, Walter and Alice, once again and meet her husband, Samuel Reed. Melissa came through the race very well. In fact, all the other Team Fox members I met—Jeremiah, Michael, Bill, Peter (whom I didn't manage to meet), and Natan—did nicely. Jeremiah's 2:35:17 was good for 16th place in his cohort of the Age Group World Championships. Vitor was up there with Jeremiah finishing in 2:31:50.

I was curious as to how Shalane Flanagan fared.

While I struggled to a personal worst of 4:55:26 in Berlin, she breezed to a 17th place finish at 2:38:32 in her first race coming out of retirement while crushing her stated three-hour finish goal. She's a wonder. In London, Shalane ran 2:35:04 to my 4:37:21.

The ratio of my finish time to hers got me thinking. I'd hoped to be somewhere closer to four hours, but this goal was becoming increasingly out of reach. In retrospect, a target finish time of four hours was inconsistent with my initial strategy. I'd rationalized that these weekly marathons should be considered as slow-paced training runs. Therefore, I should've been thinking of a 10-minute mile pace and a finish time somewhere in the ballpark of four and a half hours.

Shalane's personal goal was to complete each Major in less than three hours. Should my finish time goal be six hours; that is, twice her goal? Maybe. Perhaps a better backup goal was to finish in no more than twice Shalane's finish time. Using this contrived goal, I was already two for two. So far so good.

Definitely not one of my more aggressive objectives, but if I can finish within a factor of two of one of the greatest American marathoners, well then, I'll take that.

The morning after the race I felt good enough to take a five-mile recovery run in Hyde Park. The rest of the day was spent on a lovely trip to Worcester to visit with Steve and Louise Dunn-Massey whom Lynn and I met in Palo Alto when all our children were young. Steve and Louise moved back to the UK shortly after we met but we've stayed in touch since then. The train was Wi-Fi enabled so I took the opportunity of finishing my recap of the marathon and I posted it to my blog before pulling into the station at Worcester.

In England there are cities, towns, villages, etc. Steve explained to me that Worcester has status within England due to its cathedral, which is spectacular. Cathedrals were built centuries ago so it's virtually impossible for newer municipalities, no matter how prominent and influential they ultimately become, to gain the status of a Worcester. But I forget if that cathedral makes it a city or a town. City, perhaps? However, according to some internet search results, it appears that the United Kingdom is moving toward a new classification system determined primarily by population. Maybe this was caused by dissatisfaction amongst large communities that are too new to ever have a cathedral. I'm out of my depth here. Steve's going to have to explain all this to me again next time I see him.

⚬⚬

The next day I left London; my PCR COVID test from Boot's taken on Saturday came back negative. With the European leg completed it was off to the US where I could count on mostly uniform COVID-19 protocols if not race-related procedures. Next stop: Boston, where I would prepare for the Chicago–Boston doubleheader, the most difficult stage of this challenge.

Showtime.

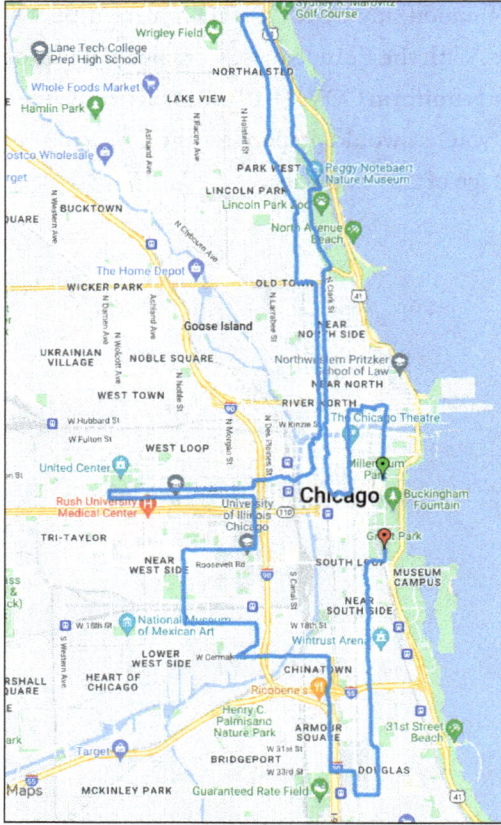
The 2021 Chicago Marathon Route (© J. Drake).

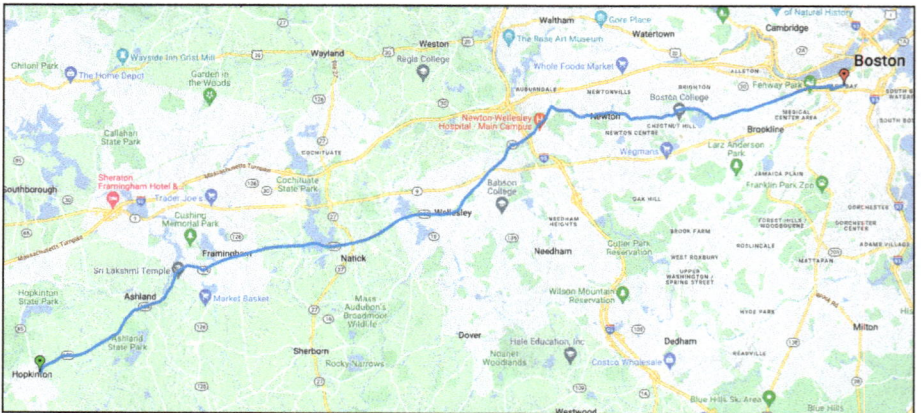
The 2021 Boston Marathon Route (© J. Drake).

13

The Doubleheader: Chicago–Boston

Lynn and I converged on Boston on Tuesday, October 5. I flew in from London while she came from Seattle bearing more Peet's and a few other running supplies that I didn't need in Europe. Lynn had booked us an Airbnb in Boston's South End just three blocks from Copley Square where the BAA was setting up camp for the marathon the following Monday. It was a convenient arrangement for getting to the Expo on Friday and to the shuttle buses for the ride to Hopkinton on race day.

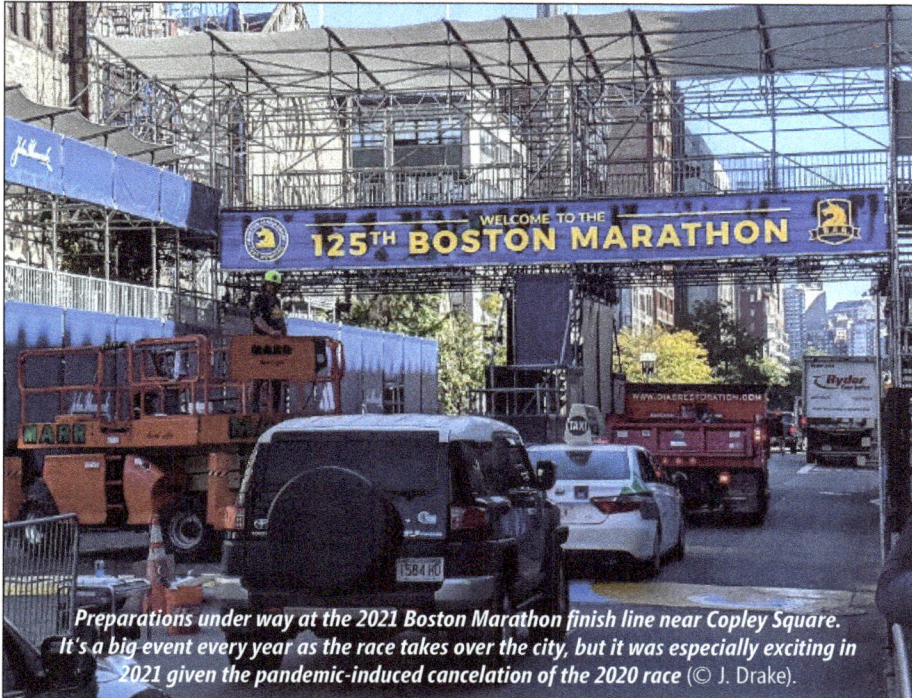

Preparations under way at the 2021 Boston Marathon finish line near Copley Square. It's a big event every year as the race takes over the city, but it was especially exciting in 2021 given the pandemic-induced cancelation of the 2020 race (© J. Drake).

I'd lived in Boston while going to university, so I knew the area well. The Boston Public Garden was only about half a mile away from the Airbnb, so I took my training runs as loops in and around it and the Common on Wednesday, Thursday, and Friday.

On Wednesday, Lynn and I met for lunch with Ed and Claire Bacher who currently live near Boston. We were introduced by our mutual friend, Larry Hyde, a neighbor from when we lived in Palo Alto, CA. Ed and Larry had run a few marathons together and Claire ran the New York City Marathon back in the 1980s. Besides having that in common, Claire also was diagnosed with Parkinson's disease a few years ago. Our feelings about exercise as an effective therapy for PD are quite similar. Unfortunately, Claire doesn't run anymore due to knee pain. Her current go-to exercise is walking.

We ate at a little French restaurant, Ma Maison, in Beacon Hill and shared stories about running, children, and our respective friendships with Larry. Lynn and I have enjoyed French cooking ever since a 1987 trip to France wherein we studied up on the genesis of the cuisine before the trip. For dessert we shared perhaps the largest profiterole that we'd ever seen. They are normally two inches or so in diameter and this one must have been at least four times that. A delicious start to my carbo loading.

Things were going to get very busy by week's end as the races approached. Hence, through Thursday I made rest a priority. Otherwise, to pass the time until then, Lynn and I did the Boston tourist thing walking about downtown, Faneuil Hall, and the South End, and eating at some lovely restaurants that Lynn selected. On Thursday, near Faneuil Hall we noticed a gentleman walking with a cane and he approached us while commenting on the London Marathon T-shirt that I was wearing from my race the previous Sunday.

He ran in London, too, and his story is astounding. His name is Bryon Solberg and he was born without a small bone called the odontoid that protects the C1 and C2 vertebrae from separating and putting pressure on the spinal cord. Most people with this condition die at an early age. Bryon is my age and he's the oldest known survivor of the disorder.

I've since done some research on Bryon and both Lynn and I have followed his exploits. He'd been an athlete his whole life but started having coordination and strength issues in 1999 when doctors discovered the condition. In 2000, he had surgery to fuse the C1 and C2 vertebrae. Between this and follow-up surgeries he had to relearn how to walk not once but twice! It was a difficult emotional adjustment for him but then he came upon the Challenged Athletes Foundation (CAF) that changed his life. Inspired by other disabled athletes he saw competing in endurance events for CAF he decided to do the same. Since then, he has run more than 100 marathons.

Honestly, you can't cast a glance about a marathon without it landing on one or more heroes.

I set aside Friday morning to visit the Expo and retrieve my race packet. COVID screening went smoothly. Boston opted for massive parallel processing, so queue times were short. Like Berlin, they went with wristbands that verified the virus status of the runner and so access to the buses and start and finish areas just involved waving the banded wrist at volunteers. COVID screening began at 9:00 am while the Expo didn't open until 11:00 am. After screening, I joined the long line of runners at the Hynes Auditorium waiting for the doors to the Expo to open.

I chatted with the lady next to me, Carita Wegner, in line to get into the Expo. Considering that this was a chance encounter, we had some eerie similarities. Both of us ran in Berlin and London the two weeks prior although she ran them both about 30 minutes faster than I did. She's a dentist and a recent transplant from the UK who'd not yet sorted through the process of setting up a practice in the US. In the meantime, like I'd done, she was considering working at a running store. She doesn't have PD but she does have a lung disease, sarcoidosis, that sounded much scarier. She actually prefers ultramarathons to marathons nowadays but couldn't pass up bagging some more Majors with this year's compressed schedule. She's working on her second pass through all the Majors and, consequently, another Six Star Medal.

Sarcoidosis is a disease wherein granulomas—tiny clumps of inflammatory cells—accumulate in one or more organs of the body.[1] The granulomas interfere with the organ's function and can eventually lead to fibrosis—the permanent scarring of organ tissue. In Carita's case, the granulomas are in her lungs but there's no guarantee that they won't spread to other organs. She was diagnosed in 2013 and she believes that running has prevented her symptoms (i.e., shortness of breath and an annoying cough) from worsening since then. Ironically, the disease pushed her from marathons into ultramarathons. Often the marathon distance is not long enough for her breathing and cough to stabilize.

It was astonishing to find out that Carita experienced the same type of benefit from endurance running that I did despite our much different ailments. In fact, with her disease the situation seemed considerably more precarious and, well, dangerous. We both know, however, that the clock is ticking and that there's no way to know how long our respective diseases will allow us to do these crazy things. So, live it up while we can. We exchanged contact information and have since remained in touch, following each other on Strava.

Race packet pickup took some time given that there were hundreds of queued runners flooding into the Expo once it opened. But there were many booths set up to handle distribution, so it went efficiently.

With my race bib secured my next objective was to get ready for Chicago and, specifically, postrace fueling. The plan had been to prepare some food in Boston to take with me to Chicago, but I never got around to that. After some thought and some internet searches I determined that chicken fried rice would be a convenient dish to purchase in Chicago for eating on the plane back to Boston. Chicken fried rice has almost the ideal 4:1 ratio of carbs to protein and would be easy to consume on the plane. I just needed to down two pounds of the stuff and I'd be all set.

Packing for the flight to Chicago didn't take long. It was just an overnighter, so I only needed the essentials: coffee, AeroPress, foam roller, running shoes and outfit, Clif Bloks, Maurten 100 Gels, Nuun tablets, toiletries, etc.

To close out Friday, Lynn and I visited with our friends, Darien Wood and Ela Barberis, and their son, Max, for a carbo-loading dinner of pasta with pesto. I'd gone to school with Darien, and now he's living in Brookline with his family. Darien has run marathons in the past, including Berlin both before and after reunification. Max is an avid high school runner. He and I worked on getting Darien to consider getting back into marathons.

Darien wouldn't commit to any more marathons, but he did commit to driving me to the airport in the morning for my flight to Chicago and to picking me up at Logan Airport upon my return Sunday night. Both he and Lynn very much wanted me to accept the offer. I stubbornly declined because I figured that I could manage those on my own since the 'T' in Boston made getting to and from Logan so convenient. I didn't want to bother Darien with that.

Lynn thought that I should reconsider arguing that, especially on the return to Boston, I'd be exhausted and could use a little help. The conversation went something like this:

Lynn: You should save your energy for Boston on Monday. After Chicago you
    will be beat. Wouldn't you want Darien to pick you up at Logan?
Me: No.

I'm a Drake, after all. Independence is in my DNA. I have a lot of practice with this.

I took an early flight from Boston that arrived at Chicago O'Hare at 11:36 am. That should've given me plenty of time to get to the Expo to pick up my race packet (to save time I'd go straight to the Expo from O'Hare with my luggage), check in at the Hilton Chicago where I would spend the night, and still make it to a Team Fox meet and greet at Elephant and Castle (E&C) that was being held from 2-4 pm. Although I wasn't a charity runner in Chicago, the folks at Team Fox invited me to join the party anyway.

This relatively uncomplicated itinerary set the tone for the 28 hours I spent in Chicago. Transit delays, long lines, and my own careless errors kept the schedule more exciting than it should've been. In the process, my self-regard as a logistics expert took a beating.

According to Google Maps, getting to the Expo from O'Hare via the 'L' trains would take me about an hour and a half. Allowing for an hour spent at the Expo picking up my race packet and perusing the exhibits, checking into the hotel by 2:30 pm seemed possible. That'd give me plenty of time to get to the Elephant and Castle on North Wabash Street before the event was over. I'd arrive well after the 2:00 pm start, but I would still have time to meet some runners and the Team Fox staff.

There was work being done on the tracks, so I was later getting to the Expo than hoped. Once there, it was clear that everyone decided to get their bibs on Saturday morning and unfortunately Chicago opted for mostly serial processing of the entrants. The line for the check-in desks didn't seem too long when I joined it, but what I couldn't see from my initial viewing point was the cavernous adjacent room (if room is the right word for something the size of at least three football fields) into which the line entered. It moved swiftly but it was extremely long, meandering haphazardly back and forth across the cavern before re-emerging at the check-in desks. Well over an hour was spent in queue to get into the Expo to retrieve my race bib.

With all that time spent at the Expo I had to hustle to get to the Elephant and Castle, so I decided to take a cab to the hotel rather than take the long walk back to the 'L.' Probably saved a little time but traffic was so snarled that I started to doubt that I'd make it to the E&C in time. I spent very little time checking in then got back to the 'L' and waited for the next train. It was a very long, frustrating wait. Somewhat relieved, at just a little before 4:00 pm I entered the sparsely populated E&C on Wabash only to find out that there was another E&C on Adams where the party was being held, as was clearly indicated on the Team Fox flyer. (Note to self: Are you sure that you have a strength in logistics and planning?) I nearly gave up at this point. I'd be getting there so late, but I chose to hoof it to the correct E&C anyway.

It was a good decision. The party was still going on and I finally had the chance to meet Liz Berger and Katie Casamassina who have been so instrumental in my getting into a number of the Majors. After hugs and photos, I sat down with a Guinness and noticed that the crowd was thinning out and I wasn't going to get a chance to meet many other runners.

However, I struck up a conversation with the Jones family at the next table and they invited me to join them. Eric was running the race on Sunday in honor of his late grandfather who had Parkinson's. He's a med student and had just started interviewing for his residency. A lot of medicine in this family. Eric's parents, Rick and Inga, are both pharmacists and his sister, Julia, is studying to become one. Julia is an accomplished runner herself but didn't run in Chicago. She, Rick, and Inga were there just to support Eric.

Meeting this family was a highlight of my adventure. They're devoted to each other and to helping eradicate PD given the many years of suffering that they witnessed in Inga's father. Eric is considering Physical Medicine and Rehabilitation (PM&R) for his specialty and is a leader in the Parkinson Association of Northern California (PANC). He's well-connected, too. For PANC's education conference later in the month Eric had lined up and would be introducing Team Fox legend Jimmy Choi as the keynote speaker.

We chatted a lot about PD and the Majors' journey that I was on. I was touched by how interested they were in my story. I found out later from Eric that after we met, the whole family started following my blog and my last entry of the series was read aloud at their dinner table. Imagine! I was blown away.

A digression here seems appropriate.

My father had Parkinson's disease and he was a runner. He'd run about a mile every morning. Some of his children would at times join him for these runs. In summer, we would often vacation on Fire Island, and I remember rising early to run with him on the beach before the hordes of sunbathers arrived.

But when I think of Dad, PD isn't the affliction that comes to mind. Rather, it was the stroke that he suffered when he was 62 that I contemplate. In fact, it may have been the stroke, or the mini-strokes that preceded it, that triggered his Parkinson's.[2] Still, it was a brain disorder that changed his life and weighed heavily on his family during his later years.

I've asked Lynn, Kinsey, and Aidan how they handled the news of my PD diagnosis. Their responses were enlightening.

They all seemed to understand, perhaps before I did, that something was amiss. Kinsey was suspicious about the foot cramps that I got while running. All of them had spotted the slight tremor in my right arm and hand. Kinsey and Aidan discussed it between themselves but not with Lynn or with me. Lynn kept the observation to herself.

It's not a subject to be broached lightly no matter how close the relationship.

Thus, when I told them of my diagnosis they were not surprised. Concerned, of course, but not surprised. They were also frightened for me. What would the future bring?

I have selfish reasons for wanting to avoid the suffering that Inga's father endured. But I also want to spare my wife and my children from having to witness it.

As the event wrapped up, I still had to get my fuel for Boston. I found a Chinese takeout restaurant and ordered some chicken fried rice to eat on the plane. With that out of the way all there was left to do was to get some sleep to prepare for a very challenging day and then wake up in time to make coffee in the hotel room while dressing for the race. The forecast was ominous; temperatures into the 70s and 80s. I needed to revise my strategy because if Chicago was a repeat of Berlin, then Boston would be nigh impossible.

During the week leading into Chicago, I pondered pacing strategies and settled on this: break up the first 24 miles into chunks of six miles each, run the first five of those at a 10-minute pace, and walk or very slow run the sixth. Repeat that sequence four times then run the last 2.2 miles with whatever I had left. This would work out to a finish time of about five hours.

I hoped that those five-mile running stretches wouldn't be too taxing in the heat and in any event the intervening slow miles would allow for cooling down, fueling, hydration, and a heartrate reset. Importantly, I figured this approach would avoid the common marathoning error of "going out too fast" because I would be reining it in to a walk after five miles. Of course, I would assess the situation constantly and dial back further if need be.

The fueling with Nuun tablets and Maurten 100 Gels worked well in London. But in irrational defiance of the "nothing new on race day" directive, after studying the on-course fueling stations in the event guide I realized that the Gatorade Endurance Formula being served may cover both my hydration and my carb needs. That Gatorade Formula was also to be served in Boston, so I thought if I could prove it out in Chicago then I could use it in Boston as well. I would carry my Nuun and Maurten, same as London, as a backup.

Another wonderful part of my association with Team Fox was that they set up headquarters for the team at Roosevelt University, very close to the start and finish lines. Food, water, gear check, luggage check, and showers were all available to us. This was a big benefit to the team, but I found it particularly useful. I checked my luggage there so that I wouldn't have to return to the hotel and with the showers provided I could clean up before heading to O'Hare.

Bill Bucklew was running in Chicago, so I caught up with him again at Roosevelt. He looked no worse for wear coming off his feats in the UK, but he admitted that he had a new issue with water retention now. I found out later from him that sweating during the race neatly took care of that for him.

We all walked the block from Roosevelt to Grant Park for the start. The organization within the park was very good. Signs and helpful, knowledgeable volunteers made it easy to find the way to the start waves. And there were far more portable toilets than in London, so the lines were only about 10 minutes long.

The atmosphere on the course was similar to Berlin and London—bands, music, wildly cheering spectators, etc. Absent were London-style costumed runners but the people of Chicago more than made up for that with copious, entertaining signage.

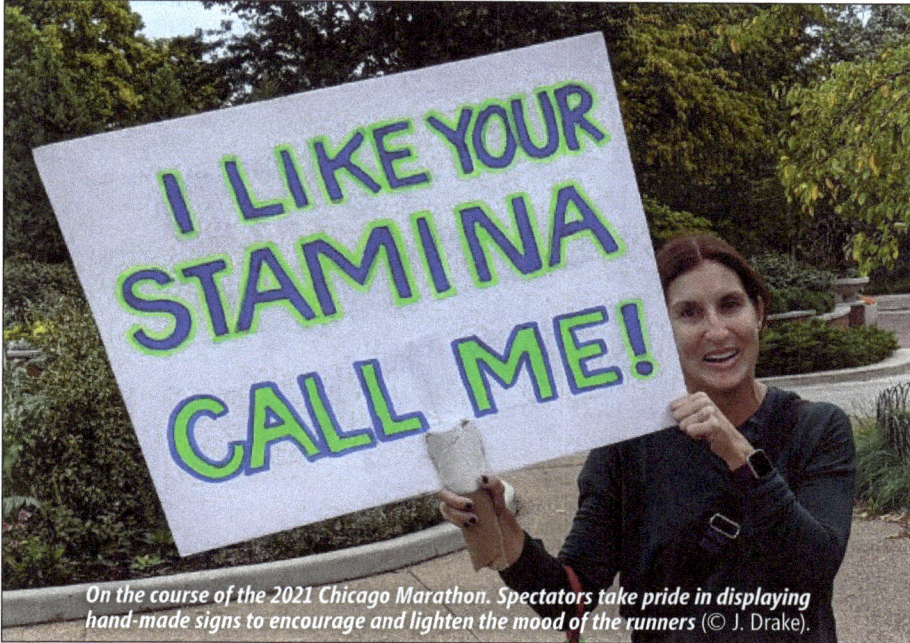

On the course of the 2021 Chicago Marathon. Spectators take pride in displaying hand-made signs to encourage and lighten the mood of the runners (© J. Drake).

A pleasant first was when, on two separate occasions, runners noted my Team Fox jersey and thanked me for raising funds for Parkinson's research as they passed by. They'd both recently lost loved ones who suffered for years with PD. I got similar props from the volunteer who handed me my finisher's medal given that his brother had just been diagnosed with PD.

Heat, humidity, and wind caused problems for many runners. I was told later that even some of the elites were suffering from the weather conditions.

My pacing strategy held up well for the first 18 miles, but the wheels fell off after that. As I thought might be the case given the conditions, I did have to rein it in toward the end. I walked some of the last miles and justified this by noting that my walking pace was not much slower than my running pace at that point and walking hurt so much less than running.

My feelings about the new fueling strategy were mixed. It could've been that the Gatorade plan worked as well as could be expected given the weather conditions, but I nonetheless felt wretched at the end of the race. As with the previous two Majors, nausea was getting to me much more than anticipated. I would need to reassess fueling for Boston.

An unplanned fueling tactic came at mile 23 when I was handed a cup of beer. That tasted very nice and, surprisingly, helped to settle my stomach.

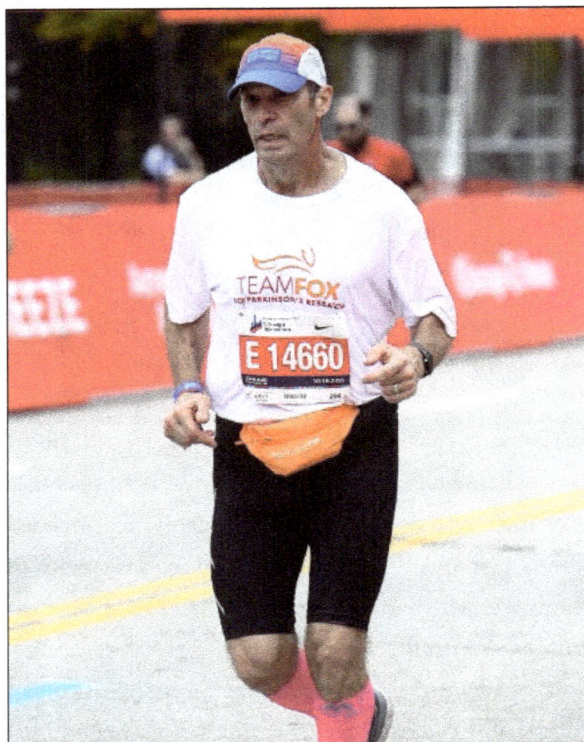

On the course in a very hot and humid 2021 Chicago Marathon.
I qualified for Chicago but ran in the Team Fox race shirt
because The Michael J. Fox Foundation was kind enough to
allow me to crash their prerace party (© J. Drake).

I brought it in at a new personal worst of 5:13:58. Bill did very well considering his exploits in his *The Long Walk* and the London Marathon beforehand. Eric is a gazelle. Despite admitting serious discomfort for much of the race he finished in 2:45:38. In fact, Eric finished in a group that included Shalane Flanagan, so he'll show up in her finish line photos and video.

Shalane finished in 2:46:38, less than 10 minutes off her London race, so if the conditions bothered her, it wasn't by much. With my 5:13:58 I was still on track with my goal of finishing within a factor of two of her time.

After the finish, I hustled back to Roosevelt University for a shower and change of clothes before my return to O'Hare Airport. Cramps in my arms, hands, back, legs, and feet were so bad that showering and dressing went painfully, painfully slow.

You will recall that I just barely made it onto my plane back to Boston. My next task was to start fueling for the next day's marathon. But some of the other passengers noticed that I'd just run the marathon, so we fell into conversation. I'm not sure what tipped them off. Maybe it was my slow shuffle to my seat and subsequent collapse into it.

I texted Lynn to let her know that I'd made the plane and that I was planning to take the 'T' back to the Airbnb after getting into Logan. She really wanted me to relent and allow her to arrange for Darien to come pick me up. Fatigue overcame my stubbornness and so I gave in. A chauffeur sounded pretty good in fact. So much for that stubborn Drake independence thing.

Across the aisle from me was Brendan Reilly who is an agent for some elite runners. He's a marathoner but he didn't run Chicago. In front of him was Jess Dorrington, a physical therapist from Portland, Oregon, who did run. We talked about how difficult the weather conditions were and Brendan noted that, with the heat, humidity, and wind, some of the elite runners had a tough time of it.

Jess and Brendan were aware that many runners were attempting both Chicago and Boston. Jess had signed up to do Boston also but ultimately decided against it. She'd done very well in Chicago (3:09:07), so I believe she found that effort to be sufficient.

I think that Jess and Brendan were both impressed with my plan to run all the Majors, same as Shalane Flanagan. Jess had related that up until this day she had run in six marathons. Brendan asked me, "How about you? How many have you run? 40?" I suppose that he thought, given the challenge that I took on, that I'd been running marathons for decades. I told him, "No, same with me, just six."

When someone wears a mask, only the eyes are available for conveying facial expressions. But reading Brendan's eyes as they fixed on mine for a beat, interpreting his brief silence, and using some imagination, I'd the impression that his jaw had dropped underneath the mask. It occurred to me that the more experienced a person is about marathons, and the closer to the elites that they dwell, the more incredulous they can be that some inexperienced unknown, like myself, would take on such a challenge.

I'm speculating here but it wouldn't surprise me if they tend to focus on the insane rigors that an elite runner suffers to prepare for their events, rigors that are out of reach for the average mortal. Recreational runners, though they are also highly respectful of the accomplishments of the elites, seem more likely to accept that anyone with the time, energy, and dedication is capable of the extraordinary, possibly because we see it all the time amongst our cohorts.

Jess, Brendan, and I exchanged names and I gave them the link to my blog. Jess told me about some awesome tools for gait analysis and other running metrics that they had at her office and suggested that I come check them out sometime. Being close to the Eugene, Oregon running mecca she knew a fair share of elite runners and had worked on and with some of them.

All this time I knew that I had to start re-fueling but my stomach wasn't game. I got a few forkfuls down but decided that I'd wait until the nausea faded. Instead, I started in on hydration and slept as much as my cramping legs would allow me.

Saint Darien collected me at Logan and dropped me off with Lynn at about 7:30 pm. It was a blessedly easy trip from the airport thanks to him and I was glad that Lynn insisted on this instead of the 'T.' One nauseated ride in a big city subway system was enough for one day.

⁓◻◻⁓

My Boston start time was 11:00 am, much more civilized than the 7:30 am Chicago start. I needn't be at the shuttle bus to Hopkinton until 9:15 am, and the walk to the Boston Common where I'd meet the bus would take me maybe 20 minutes.

That gave me something like 13 hours to prepare for Boston. I slept as well as I could, but my leg cramps were still raging making rest hard to come by. Between intermittent naps I worked on the Chicago recap for my blog and finished off the rest of the chicken fried rice. In fact, my appetite had returned so I ate pretty much everything else we had on hand as well.

Though I was fairly certain that my followers would've been understanding, I didn't want them to have to wait another day for my blog update. They continued to follow me closely, some of them texting or emailing me a few hours before the start of each race, and it seemed only fair to keep them informed in real time. Besides, I'd grown into my role as a storyteller and from a narrative point of view it didn't make sense to me to have them follow along with my Boston effort without getting the Chicago details first. At about 2:00 am, I published the Chicago recap.

By 5:00 am my leg cramps finally subsided, and I was able to get some rest before having some coffee, suiting up for the race, kissing Lynn goodbye, and heading out for the shuttle buses.

Boston did a rolling start in Hopkinton. Runners were loaded onto the buses in wave start order and once deposited in Hopkinton they simply walked the three-quarters of a mile to the start line, stopping to use the portable toilets as needed along the way. Chip timing allows runners to decide for themselves when to cross the starting line to begin their race. All the other races had chip timing, too, but these other races opted for mass corral starts and announcements before each wave was launched. Boston's was a decidedly more relaxed approach.

Just before I started my race, I got an unexpected boost. I'd missed the Team Fox prerace dinner due to my appointment in Chicago, so I wasn't able to meet the rest of the runners beforehand. But at the starting line one of them, Alexis, realized who I was from the Team Fox jersey I wore and gave me a big hug to get my day off to a great start.

My pacing strategy for the race was modified from the day before. I was still fatigued from Chicago, so I expected an overall slower pace in Boston. Yet, the first half of the Boston course was mostly downhill, so I was hoping to coast through that without resorting to the run/walk strategy of Chicago. It was a few degrees cooler than Chicago, too, so that helped. Very important, though, this time around there were several groups of supporters along the route planning to cheer for me as I passed. They were positioned at miles 14, 20, and 24, and, of course, there would be hundreds of Wellesley women out near mile 13. I wanted to look my best at all of these stations. Any necessary walk breaks would need to be timed and executed wisely.

As was the case in Berlin, London, and Chicago, the spectators were fantastic in Boston. It was a party along the whole route just like for the other races, but Boston put on its own spin.

Like early on when a dozen or so mini-trampolines were placed curbside along the route. Some runners stopped to do a few giddy bounces before heading off again.

And "Sweet Caroline" (ba ba ba!) was the clear favorite for music along the route.

Some spectators offered alternative fueling strategies to the runners. Promising approaches that I sampled along the way included pretzels, Oreo cookies, salt, and orange slices.

These marathons have highlighted for me the work I need to do on fueling and hydration to be better prepared for any future races. Again, my preference for carrying a hydrations vest was not allowed. I decided that the Gatorade from Chicago was not better than the Nuun/Maurten combination that I used in London, so I reverted to the earlier strategy.

My stomach became unsettled once again midway through the race, so I'd no strong desire to slurp down the rest of my Maurten supply. Instead, as needed, I grazed on the pretzels and Oreos. The Oreos felt like comfort food for my gut. I'm now seriously considering them as a mainstay for my future fueling needs due to their medicinal value.

It started off pretty well. Despite being beaten up in Chicago and still rather sluggish I managed a reasonable, albeit slow, pace for the first 15 miles. The downhill slope of the first few miles certainly helped. By the halfway mark I was only about eight minutes off of what I'd done in Chicago.

Then I got my first on-course pick-me-up at just before the halfway mark. On the spot, I worked out the solution to the Wellesley Scream Tunnel. In hindsight it should've been obvious and though it may've occurred to other runners I didn't see it employed at the time. As I ran by, I blew, and received, countless noncontact, socially distant kisses to the apparent delight of the ladies lining the course.

Shortly afterward I came upon the mile 14 Team Fox cheer section where Liz Diemer led the raucous cheering as they saw me approach from far off and kept up the noise until I passed. The noise, the high fives, and the photo-taking made for an unforgettable and unexpected emotional rush.

Then the rolling hills of Newton began. It had warmed up considerably and my heartrate spiked above 160 bpm. I chose to walk mile 16 then picked up the pace again for miles 17 through 21, running well enough to look respectable at the second Team Fox cheer section at mile 20. That one was joined by my university friend, Dave Plummer, and again I got a much-needed lift from all the cheering and high fives.

The heat took its toll, and the crash came at the end of mile 21. I had to slow to a walk for fear of passing out. It took nearly two miles of walking for my lightheaded staggering to recede. Then at Coolidge Corner, about mile 24, Darien, Ela, and Max, gave me the final emotional shove I needed to get me "running" again for the last two or so miles to the finish.

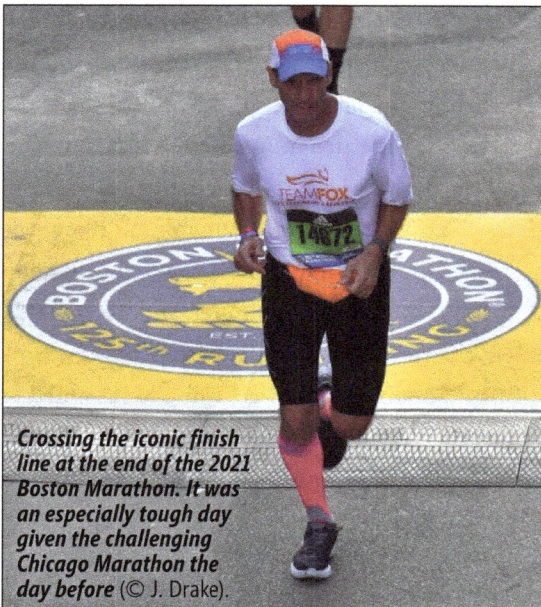

Crossing the iconic finish line at the end of the 2021 Boston Marathon. It was an especially tough day given the challenging Chicago Marathon the day before (© J. Drake).

Lynn and our friend, Joanna Forbes, positioned themselves on Boylston Street close to the end. They cheered mightily but I didn't hear or notice them, as I was so focused on crossing the finish line.

One surreal, made for TV moment happened toward the end of the race that I only learned of afterward. Friends and family on both coasts were using the race's app to track my progress and a glitch made it look as if I'd stopped cold at 40 kilometers[3] (slightly under 25 miles) with less than two miles to go.

Lynn was deluged with "Oh no, what happened?" texts. I think that my selfie post to Facebook wearing the finisher's medal put an end to the drama.

Team Fox hosted a postrace dinner from 4-6 pm but I finished at nearly 4:30 and with cleaning up and a little rest time I wasn't able to make that one either. I regretted that considering how much I enjoyed all the other meet and greets held by Team Fox, but my body wasn't cooperating. Aaron, Max, Alexis, and Eric all did well on the day.

Instead, after a little down time, Lynn and I chose to convene later with Darien and his family in Brookline along with some other friends who were nearby. Steve Potter and Hauke-Kite Powell and his partner, Arlene, joined us as did Dave and Joanna who had cheered for me along the course. It was so great to see everyone. Once again, the show of support was energizing. It gave me the strength and motivation to regale them with tales from all the Majors that I'd run to date. I also reminded them that I hoped to return in April 2022 for the next Boston Marathon and suggested that we do all this again at that time.

Shalane finished in 2:40:34 thus improving on a difficult day in Chicago by more than six minutes. I lumbered in at 5:24:34, yet another new personal worst, and missed my factor of two goal by 3 minutes and 26 seconds. I was forced to admit that I'm not half the runner that Shalane is.

The Chicago–Boston doubleheader was difficult. As noted earlier, training in the cool climate of Seattle had given me a false sense of security that was exposed when I ran in hotter weather. Although I was aware of my sensitivity to the heat, I had no idea of the toll that it could take.

Parkinson's surely is influential here. One common symptom of PD is heavy sweating and I do indeed sweat profusely making me more susceptible to dehydration. Getting the hydration right during a marathon, with the correct electrolyte amount, is a critical factor for me in hot and humid weather.

All in all, though, not too shabby. The hardest part of the quest was over and only two more marathons remained to be conquered: Seattle (as the virtual stand-in for Tokyo) and New York City. Both would be at temperatures more to my liking than Berlin, Chicago, and Boston. Granted, I had only six days to prepare for Seattle but then I had three languid weeks before NYC.

I felt fortunate to escape from these four races without any serious damage to the power train: feet, legs, knees, hips. I was sore, of course, but that's no problem. I can run sore. It's a far cry from a stress fracture or joint inflammation that might have derailed the whole show. And though I had some back troubles in Europe, the beds in the US weren't causing me any issues so far. As Lynn and I left Boston I was feeling pretty good about completing this challenge.

My Virtual Tokyo–Seattle Marathon Route (© J. Drake).

14

Tokyo aka Seattle

My luck ran out on our flight back to Seattle.

It started with a sore throat. By nightfall it was a full-on cold and the next two days I was wiped out and bedridden except for the time I took to get tested—it wasn't COVID.

Being in bed for so long brought on my chronic back issue. By Saturday, October 16, the day before I planned to run the virtual substitute for the Tokyo Marathon, I was still shaking off the lingering cold and my capricious back made for painful walking.

All the COVID-safe protocols in Chicago and Boston should've protected me from contagion. It makes me wonder how a cold got through all that. Maybe it had something to do with running mile after mile amidst thousands of others through city streets lined with tens of thousands of additional spectators. Perhaps someone coughed near me in the airport. Or maybe it was from being packed inside a tightly sealed aircraft. I'll never know.

By bedtime October 16, running a marathon the next day was borderline folly. But then, what part of this whole campaign hadn't been?

Virtual road races came on strong in 2020 as the pandemic disrupted social gatherings of all sorts. The process is familiar: the runner registers for the race, pays an entry fee, runs the race, and collects a T-shirt and perhaps a medal for the effort. The difference with a virtual race is that there's no start or finish line and, usually, no pack of runners to run with. Instead, the runner simply runs wherever and whenever he wants for the prescribed distance and then logs the finish time to the race's online results page. T-shirts and/or medals are shipped to the runner's home. Typically, there's a specific date window during which the race must be run.

Although it's possible for a runner to compare her results to others, places and standings aren't so meaningful given that each runner may run a unique course.

To soften the blow of the cancellation and/or downsizing of the in-person events, in 2020 all of the Majors held virtual marathons with fewer, if any, restrictions regarding who may register; that is, qualification standards no longer applied. However, the virtual versions of the races don't count toward achieving a Six Star Medal.

Many runners, including myself, found the virtual races to be an acceptable if not entirely satisfying outlet for the substantial training they'd been doing for races that were summarily canceled. I personally ran a 5K, two 10Ks, a 15K, two half marathons, and one marathon virtually in 2020.

Despite the return of the in-person events, race coordinators continue to find a place for the virtual races. It helps to offset the high demand for some of the races that're hard to get into. By augmenting the in-person race with a virtual one, for example, the 2021 London Marathon promoted a worldwide event with 35,300 runners on the streets of the city joined by another 24,000 running in venues all around the world. It appears that London will continue to make the virtual race an annual fixture.

Tokyo, having postponed its marathon to March 6, left runners only the virtual option for the scheduled October 17 race.

In spite of my cold and my aching back, I was loathe to stray from the schedule I set for my Virtual Tokyo Marathon. Thus, on the morning of October 17, after coffee, successful albeit painful contortions to don my compression socks, and feeling at maybe 70% capable, I decided to go for it. At worst I would call it off midway and make it up some other day. I had no finish time pressure; if it took six hours to complete, so be it.

I chose a course like one I've used for some of my 20-mile-long runs. Using roads and trails along the perimeter of West Seattle, it's replete with breathtaking Puget Sound and downtown Seattle views. I threw in a few loops around Lincoln Park to top off the distance to 26.2 miles.

My first few strides weren't promising. Each jarring footfall sent a surge of pain to my lower back. Nonetheless, I headed for Lincoln Park hoping that it'd loosen up with a few more miles.

At the park I met up with Mike Marshino and Erika Whinihan, two gazelles that I've befriended on Strava after meeting them through working at West Seattle Runner. They both ran Boston and turned in finish times well over an hour faster than mine. Erika ran it in 3:31:41 and Mike finished in 3:16:02.

Mike enjoys travel. Following him on Strava, in recent months I've seen him post runs from Hawaii, New York City, Las Vegas, San Diego, and so on. He often meets up with his dad on these trips and they'll do a half marathon together.

Erika joined me for a few miles in the park kindly throttling back her pace for my benefit and gave me much-needed encouragement as I plodded along still hoping for my back to thaw out. We chatted about how Boston went for each of us and about just stuff in general. Introvert that I am, I rarely run with a partner but this time it was very pleasant to have Erika to shoot the breeze with. Took my mind off of my back pain.

Erika is one of those runners with an insane amount of energy. Besides being a mom, she works as a business manager at Microsoft while she's attending graduate school at the University of Washington studying to be a librarian. She often posts her training runs to Strava at 5:00 am. I'm in awe.

At the halfway mark, well after Erika peeled off for home, things weren't going much better with my back. Then at about mile 17 the miracle that I was hoping for came through. The ache vanished and my pace picked up to sub 10 minutes per mile and I was able to sustain that through the end of the race. As Lori McConnell of West Seattle Runner quipped, "Nothing like the moment when endorphins cancel out the pain."

I finished the second half a full 17 minutes faster than the first. No walking, no cramps, and no wall. Undoubtedly, the relative coolness (the temperature was 53 degrees) made a huge difference. My overall time was no great shakes, but it wasn't another personal worst and it was enormously gratifying to put this one in the books.

But the real thrill was that on this lonely, mostly solo run I actually had spectators rooting for me! When passing Constellation Park at mile 17.5 there were signs urging me on placed by my neighbors, Owen and Amy Reese, and their son, Milo. George and Beth Riddell were there as well cheering for me as I passed. It was as energizing, if not more so, as any of the cheering that I heard at the in-person marathons I'd just run.[1]

My route took me further around Alki Point then I doubled back to finish upon return to Constellation Park. Everyone was still there at the end as was Jim Bergstrom, cheering from his balcony overlooking the scene. I couldn't have asked for a better day than this one.

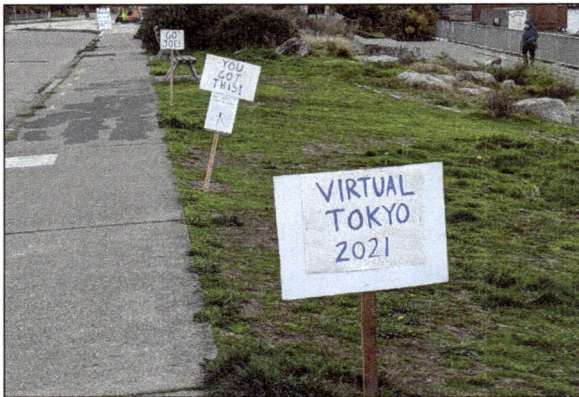

My very own personal "finish line" signage displayed during my Virtual Tokyo Marathon in West Seattle (© J. Drake).

I knew from history that this bout with my back wasn't over. The relief that I felt during the latter half of the race was to be temporary. Plus, I hadn't fully recovered from my cold. I needed another four days of rest afterward before I was able to get back to training for New York City. I put together a recap and published it to my blog the day after the virtual race.

I looked for some report about how Shalane fared in her virtual that she planned to do in her hometown of Portland, Oregon but there was nothing on October 17. She ended up doing what I probably should've done and ran it the following day, Monday, October 18. Her finish time was 2:35:14 to my 4:41:55. So after failing to meet my factor of two objective in Boston, I was back on track.

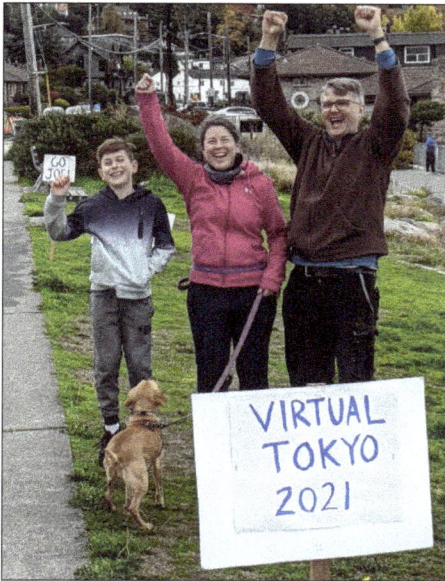

Milo, Amy, and Owen Reese, cheering for me as I finished the virtual marathon that I ran in Seattle in place of the 2021 Tokyo Marathon that had been rescheduled for March 6, 2022 (© J. Drake).

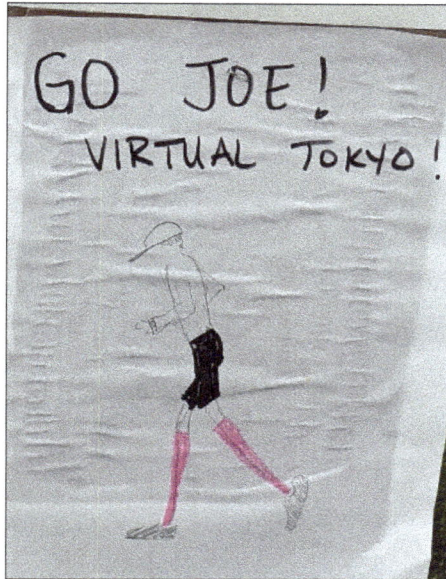

Amy Reese came up with this sign to display while I ran my virtual marathon in West Seattle. It neatly captures my preferred race attire. The drawing ultimately became the inspiration for this book's cover art created by my sister, Patricia Snyder (© J. Drake).

15

Team 50

It'd been a two-year crash course in marathon running and as the final 2021 World Marathon Major in New York City loomed, this stage of the adventure was coming to an end. I'd spent a lot of time researching best practices and integrating them into my training strategy. Perhaps with some changes I might've performed better but, on the whole, I'm satisfied with how prepared I was.

One thing that I wasn't prepared for that continues to amaze me is the tacit and unbridled support that runners have for each other. It's so unlike other, particularly American, environments where trash talk and intentional divisiveness run amok.

Intrinsically, marathon runners acknowledge that theirs is not a zero-sum game. One runner's success in no way diminishes the achievements of others. All efforts are celebrated.

This may not be the case for the elites where there're only so many podium positions and, for example, a very limited number of Olympic berths to compete for. I couldn't say for sure having never been in that position. But for the overwhelming majority of us, the atmosphere is one of mutual, generous support.

It's not just fellow runners who promote this environment. Race directors, municipalities, volunteers, and spectators to say nothing of friends and family, are all aligned to help bring out the best performances from each athlete.

Think of it as institutionally supported audacity. It's no wonder that under these conditions individuals shrug off obstacles and their own limitations to say, effectively, "I belong here. I can do this."

The organization that puts on the New York City Marathon, New York Road Runners (NYRR), gets it. Their mission is to help and inspire people through running. To demonstrate this in a big way, and to commemorate the 50th edition of their marathon, NYRR announced *Team 50*, an impressive group of runners in their 2021 marathon.

The NYRR Public Relations team had the daunting task of selecting *Team 50* from among the 30,000 entrants. A member of the PR team, Laura Paulus, herself a runner, shared with me the team's point of view that on marathon day it's about much more than just the running. The composition of *Team 50* reflects this.

Here are just a few *Team 50* members who I found to be particularly audacious (the full list of *Team 50* members can be found on NYRR's website under Media Center):[1]

- In 2020, *Chris Nikic* became the first athlete with Down Syndrome to complete an Ironman triathlon. In 2021, he added the Boston Marathon to his accomplishments and, less than three weeks later, he ran in NYC. He's using his newly earned stardom to help dispel the stigma associated with people having physical and intellectual disabilities.

- *Aaron Lee Burros* was shot five times while saving the lives of three of his coworkers during a workplace shooting. Formerly an ultramarathoner, Aaron now struggles with shorter distances due to lingering effects of his wounds. Undeterred, going into the NYC Marathon, he was in the process of raising $50,000 for the St. Jude Children's Hospital while running 50 marathons in 50 states over the course of 50 weeks.

- *Zahra* escaped Afghanistan five days before it fell to the Taliban. Though she ran three marathons in Afghanistan before the fall, women have since been banned from sports and from educational opportunities. She ran in NYC with the charity, Free to Run, which enables women and girls to engage in outdoor activity in conflict-affected regions.

- *Sara Zutter* is a special education teacher and children's running coach in New York City who encourages her students to keep their hearts healthy. She speaks from experience having been diagnosed with atrial fibrillation and undergoing heart surgery at age 30. The surgery gave her a second chance to realize her goals of completing all six of the Marathon Majors and of competing in triathlons. Then in 2019, she was diagnosed with uterine myoma, polyps, menorrhagia, and anemia. While training for the NYC Marathon she had the myoma and polyps removed yet still raced and, in the process, raised awareness about heart disease and reproductive system disorders.

- *Micaela (Mica) Naibryf* and *Amnon Liebowitz* ran together to honor the memory of Mica's brother, Ilan, who died in the Champlain Towers collapse in Surfside, Florida. Ilan was in town to attend the funeral of a friend's father and spent the fateful night in the Towers. Amnon is a structural engineer from Israel brought in to assist with disaster relief and was the one who recovered Ilan's body.

Shalane Flanagan, the race's 2017 champion, and I made the team for running all the World Major Marathons in 2021. Shalane was highlighted for completing each of them in under three hours while I was mentioned for Parkinson's and for raising money for The Michael J. Fox Foundation as a member of Team Fox.

It's difficult to feel worthy of the juxtaposition but, nevertheless, I was delighted and honored to have my name associated with these heroes.

Laura and her colleague at NYRR Public Relations, Samantha Miller, sourced out my story to the media. They set up interviews with *Runner's World* and *The Seattle Times* and a live interview with the new streaming *Fox Weather* channel on Friday evening, two days before the race in NYC.

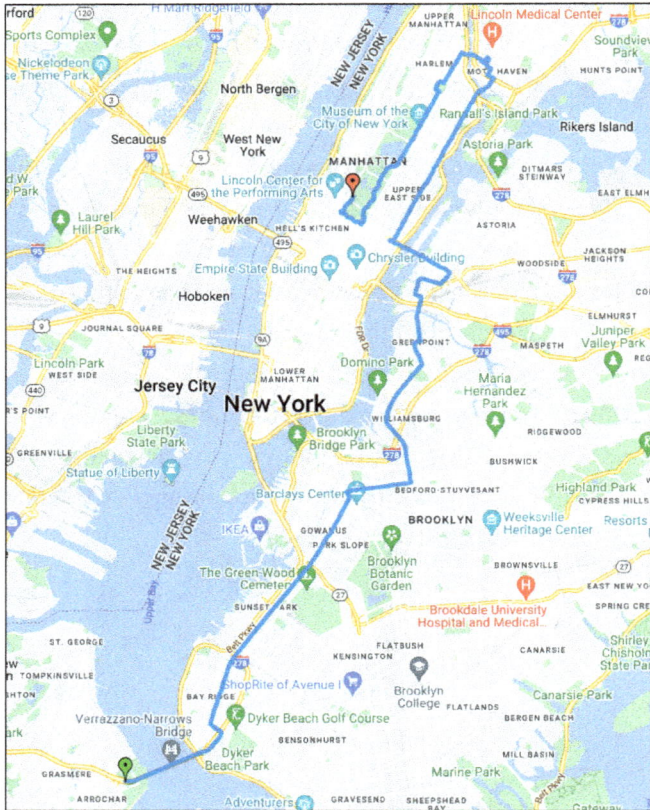

The 2021 New York City Marathon Route (© J. Drake).

16
New York City

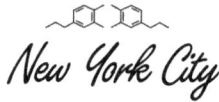

News of my Marathon Majors challenge spread since my *Team 50* designation and that led to the inevitable comparisons. Interviewers asked, "Which of these races was your favorite?"

The question came up even before I had the benefit of running in New York City and so I didn't have all the information to allow for a comprehensive answer. Up until NYC, I had the most fun in Boston because I'd friends there to cheer me on. That factor easily overwhelmed the fatigue that I carried over from Chicago the day before.

Notwithstanding, my answer to the interviewers was that I expected NYC to be the best because so many runners I'd met during the prior weeks raved about it. New York spectators had the reputation for being the most awesome of any of them and I was really looking forward to that. Furthermore, the throngs would include some of my family coming in from Long Island where I grew up. And importantly, the weather forecast called for a nearly ideal temperature of 51 degrees during the race.

It turned out that I was right about NYC being the best. But as has been the case many times during this journey, the details would surprise me.

For New York City, Lynn booked us another great Airbnb a few blocks from Central Park. I would take my training runs there and the walk back from the finish of the race promised to be short. It was, however, a four-flight walkup. That might be an issue postrace but until then, not a problem.

Our schedule in New York City was full. MJFF has its headquarters there and with a large allocation of runners in the race, Team Fox made a big deal of it.

We were invited to several events to be held at their headquarters on 33rd Street between 6th and 7th Avenues, including the traditional meet and greet for runners on Saturday, the eve of the race. They were also holding a postrace celebration at a restaurant named Stout. I learned my lesson from Chicago and double-checked: there were indeed multiple Stouts in NYC, so I confirmed that the one to go to was the Stout near 6th Avenue and 39th Street.

Also, Laura Paulus invited us to some NYRR activities at the finish area in Central Park Friday afternoon. That was an opportunity to meet with other *Team 50* runners and to work through some details with the media outreach that Laura initiated.

I'm one of 12 children and many of my siblings were coming into NYC to cheer for me. We'd be meeting at our Airbnb on Saturday evening before the race. Our mother is in an assisted-living facility way out on the eastern end of Long Island, so I planned to take the opportunity on Monday morning after the race to visit with her.

Lynn, my daughter, Kinsey, and I met up with Laura Paulus at the Marathon Kickoff activities in Central Park later on Friday.* I also met with Samantha Miller who arranged my interactions with journalists. Samantha gave me the scoop on what to expect with the *Runner's World* and *The Seattle Times* interviews, which we set up for Monday morning while I'd be out on Long Island. I also had several preparatory phone calls with the *Fox Weather* staff for the live streaming interview later that evening.

At the kickoff, NYRR had staged a few youth-runner related events. Some 400 kids participated in the "Run with Champions," a short race from 86th Street to the marathon finish line. Shalane Flanagan was on hand to pass out medals to the kids. There was also a presentation of a $75,000 donation by Abbott World Marathon Majors to NYRR youth programs on Shalane's behalf for running the six 2021 World Marathon Majors.

I did manage to meet up with Shalane when the media hordes allowed. She was kind and gracious, but I don't believe that she was aware of anyone else attempting

---

* My son, Aidan, was unable to join us on this trip due to his job in Seattle. However, he'd been following my progress closely all along and sent his love and encouragement before and after each race.

the same feat that she was. When I told her what I was doing, she said, "We should have joined forces." Awesome.

I'd some reservations about doing the *Fox Weather* spot but, after doing some research, I was happy to find that *Fox Weather* is not like *Fox News*. *Fox Weather*, though clearly seeking to entertain, is not opposed to science and had previously aired serious segments related to climate change. *Fox Weather*, of course, is in no way related to Team Fox.

Originally, they pitched to me the idea that I would report on how the weather effects a marathoner's performance. Because, like, it's a weather program. But that didn't actually come up in the interview and the focus was more about a runner doing six marathons in six weeks despite having Parkinson's. The hosts, Nick Kosir and Marissa Torres, were very pleasant to talk to and were well-briefed on my exploits. I tried to make up for my lack of prior TV experience by smiling a lot and being polite to my hosts.

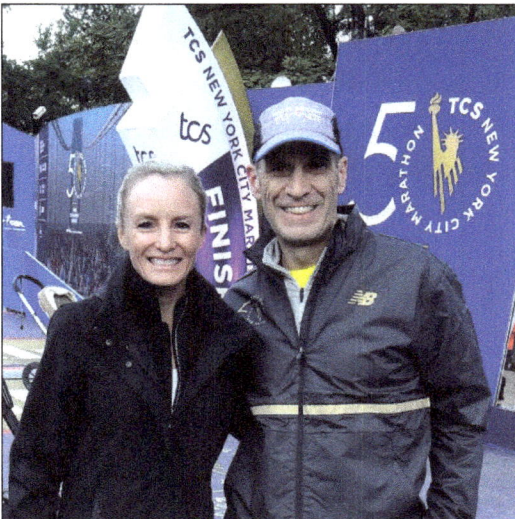

Though we had been to all of the same marathons (save the virtual ones) Shalane Flanagan and I did not cross paths until New York City. Here we are together at the 2021 New York City Marathon finish line the day before the race (© K. Drake).

Nick, by the way, has some internet fame as *The Dancing Weatherman*. I looked up some of his dance videos and he's pretty good. I was hoping he might bust a few moves during our segment but, alas, that didn't happen.

The *Fox Weather* team sent me a clip afterward so I have an idea of how I came across. I'll keep that to myself but I did thoroughly enjoy the attention.

Saturday afternoon was spent at the Team Fox meet and greet. MJFF headquarters is in a fantastic location that brings back childhood memories of *Miracle on 34th Street* and trips to the city on Thanksgiving morning to watch the parade. Looking out the window is a view of Macy's; MJFF staffers often come to the office on Thanksgiving Day to watch from on high above blimp level.

Team Fox has a large presence in the NYC Marathon where I believe they provide more than 50 entries to runners. So, there were many people to meet at the headquarters on Saturday. I didn't get to meet everyone but I was quite happy to cross paths again with Liz D., Liz B., Katie, and others from London, Chicago, and Boston. Such wonderful people—big hugs and kudos to me for my races so far.

I also spent some time talking to Dorothea Donelan Avery, her mom, Maureen, and her friend, Sue Bilotta, who is on the MJFF Board of Directors. Dorothea was running in NYC and seemed concerned about the race the next day. She needn't have worried, she did fine, finishing several minutes faster than I did.

At the event runners were adorning their names to their race jerseys using iron-on letters. I decided to do the same choosing to use pink letters to match the pink compression socks I planned to wear.

Afterward I headed back to the Airbnb to meet up with family. Lynn and Kinsey were there along with brothers Tom and Bob, and sisters Charlotte, Christine, Marcia, and Pat. Tom brought his wife, Sue, and Christine brought her daughter, Samantha. We spent the evening carbo loading on pizza and beer and plotted our respective strategies for marathon day. It was to be a busy one. There was the race of course, which would go on most of the day, and then afterward we were headed for the Team Fox postrace party at Stout.

New York City had an efficient twist to race packet pick-up. Each runner was asked to reserve a one-hour time slot for their visit to the Expo thus huge crowds were avoided. I had my bib and finisher's shirt within 10 minutes of arriving. And all the volunteers at the Expo, on the course, and at the start were friendly, professional, and helpful.

I would have preferred, though, to have the bus to the starting line deposit me on Staten Island a little closer to my start time. Not sure why the bus was scheduled to depart so early—5:15 am for a 10:00 am start. A later bus would've meant a more leisurely cup of coffee. I was warned of this by other runners but, still, I couldn't help but think that the four hours of shivering that I did leading up to the start was eating significantly into my glycogen stores. The very early arrival meant no lines at the toilets, so that was a plus.

I passed the time chatting with Tess Newland, an MBA student at the Booth Business School in Chicago. She was running in her first marathon and had a very healthy, whatever-happens-I'm-good attitude about it. In fact, she was well-prepared. She predicted a finish in 4:30:00 and ended up at 4:43:12.

All the races arrange for some kind of escort for the elite runners. This helps to protect them from the crowds while also providing valuable on-the-spot information as to the position and separation of the lead runners. In New York City the escort is provided by well-trained bicyclists.

My brother, Bob, has been a bicycle escort for the marathon for years now. Pretty cool to have him performing that critical role only just a few hours ahead of where I was pounding the pavement.

As was the case with all the Majors, hundreds of thousands of locals turned out to fire up the runners. Team Fox set up three cheer stations on the course. I didn't spot the one in Brooklyn at about mile 7, but I understand that I was seen by them yet was oblivious to their rallying cries.

Maybe that was due to the distraction caused by the overall awesomeness of the spectators lining the course. I wore my name on my shirt, courtesy of the iron-on at MJFF headquarters, and throughout the race I was urged along with a steady stream of "You got this, Joe," "I see you, Joe. Looking good," "Keep it up, Joe, almost there," and so on. It was as if all the spectators were on the course expressly to help me along.

As advertised, cooler temperatures prevailed. That was a welcome gift and I was still going at a relatively strong pace coming up to the second Team Fox station on 1st Avenue and 86th Street (about mile 17.5). Strong, that is, until I crested 86th and came upon the sight that nearly stopped me in my tracks, at first made me smile, and very nearly made me cry.

My family made up eight 'Joe Heads' (larger than life-sized photographs of my face attached to yardsticks) and were displaying them merrily as I approached the cheer station. Apparently, Marcia had enlisted Lynn's help with the planning but I'd no idea.

I slowed down long enough to give high fives to everyone and I hope I managed to choke out how awesome they all were. Then off I went toward the Bronx wishing someone would hand me a tissue.

The inevitable wall came at mile 21 and I decided to walk mile 22. Knowing that there was another Team Fox/Team Drake cheer station coming up at 5th Avenue and 93rd (about mile 23.5), I felt that a short rest would help me to look good for this next one.

As planned, my family and friends moved over to 5th Avenue in time for my arrival, but this time there was no way I was going to pass by without stopping to take a photo. It's a classic destined to live on in Drake lore for generations.

I was prepared for the second 'Joe Head' forest, so the emotion was not as moist as I headed into Central Park with nearly three miles to go. These last few miles were tough. I really wanted to finish strong but I wasn't feeling it. I slowed to a walk just shy of the 25-mile mark.

And then the photographers showed up.

At most marathons, race photographers are sprinkled about the entire route so that afterward each runner has dozens of photos to commemorate the event. But *Runner's World* has their own contract photographers that they use for the articles they write.

I knew that this was going to happen and even had Samantha Miller send them a photo of me in one of my other races so that they'd know what I looked like. Naively, I thought that this would be something like a few shots of me as I ran by.

That is not how it's done. As I came into view, the photographer would set up for some shots then as I got close, he'd turn around and sprint up ahead to set up for some more shots. Certainly, I didn't want to be walking in these photos. I picked up the pace so that, once again, I would look good for the camera. And smiles only, please. No need to advertise the pain I felt.

The first photographer stalked me in this manner for about half a mile and seemed to get his fill. We high fived and then he left and I figured that was that; I could relax a bit to the finish. I had understood that *Runner's World* was only sending one photographer to capture me on the course.

Then I came up on another photographer starting at about a half mile from the finish line. His job it seemed was to track me all the way to the end. Same deal: suck it up, look good for the cameras, repeat.

Actually, I'm grateful for their work. Because of them I finished faster than I would have otherwise and no doubt looked better doing it. The second one, Johnny Zhang, stayed long enough to document my receiving the medal. By the time he was done, though I ached, I was feeling pretty good about the whole day. Thinking

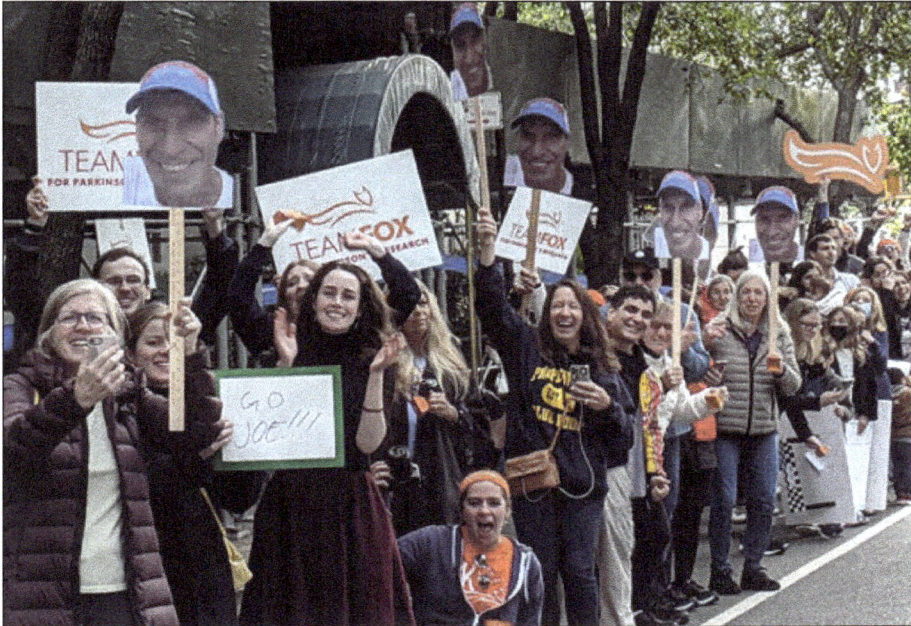

This is the Team Fox cheer station on 5th Avenue and 93rd. I stopped during the race to snap this photo. My wife, Lynn, is to the far left taking a photo of me at the same time. My family and friends are holding the 'Joe Heads' that I saw for the first time at the earlier Team Fox cheer station on 1st Avenue and 86th (© J. Drake).

back on it, it's strange that they needed two photographers. One should've been enough. And maybe it was only Johnny that *Runner's World* sent because his photo credits were the ones I saw in the article when it was published. I didn't get the other guy's name; I may never know who sent him.

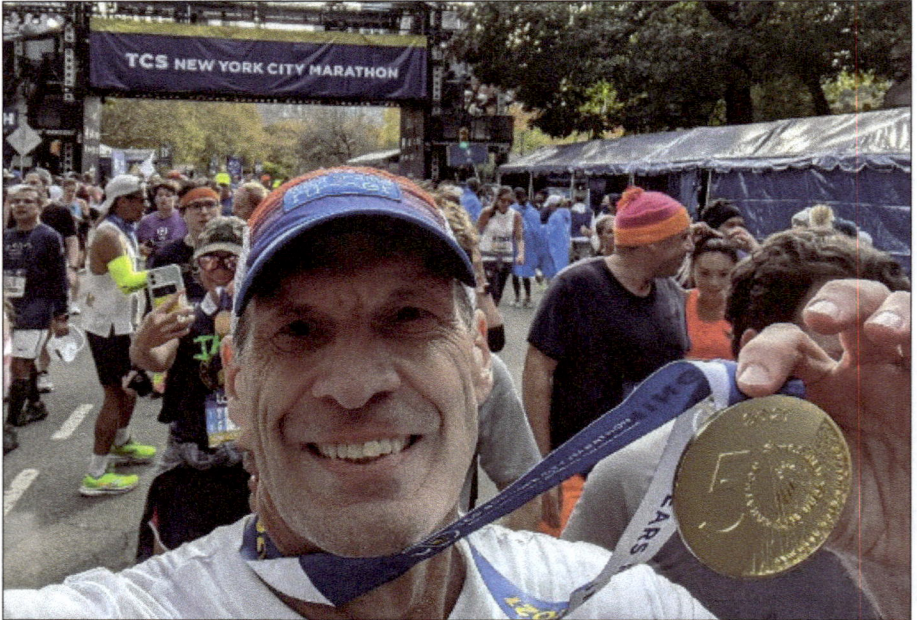

The end of the road. At the finish of the sixth and final marathon in New York City. Six marathons in 43 days, including all the Majors that I could get into (Berlin, London, Chicago, Boston, and New York City). Take that Parkinson's and shove it (© J. Drake).

Shortly after finishing I sought out a pretzel stand and bought one. I had heeded John Porter's suggestion that he gave to me when we were in Berlin—carry $20 during the race so that I could do just this as a reward for finishing.

The elation at the finish line took a disquieting turn as I made my way back to the Airbnb. It should have been a short walk. As the crow flies my return path was less than a mile eastward across the park but due to crowd control and road closures my trip home took more than an hour as I was shunted westward then forced south to give the park, and other runners still on the course, a wide berth.

Yet, even this death march turned out to have a surprisingly enjoyable angle. My finisher's poncho gave me away and so random folks would shower me with congratulations, smiles, thumbs up, and what have you as I trudged along. When did New Yorkers become so pleasant?

There were millions of them, it seems, taking the time to enjoy the event. But what will always astound me is the number of family and friends who saw fit to take part. I should note that this was a big turnout for my siblings; more than half of us were there, a percentage that I usually only see at weddings. Kinsey had brought along her friend, Janet Titzler, to help out at the Team Fox cheer stations and she also enlisted her friend, Eric Foelsch, currently living in Brooklyn, to look out for me. We missed each other but touched base by text afterward. In a last-minute appearance, our friend, Rich Mastrangelo, bicycled in from New Jersey to join in. And there were many, many others in Europe and on both coasts tracking my progress from home.

The merrymaking extended beyond the race. The 'Joe Head' prop was a big hit. I've seen countless photos of 'Joe Heads' popping up all over the city: 'Joe Head' on the subway, 'Joe Head' in a floral display stopping to smell the roses, 'Joe Head' being interviewed by a local TV crew, random parents of other runners cradling 'Joe Heads,' musicians dancing with 'Joe Heads,' etc. You get the picture. My family knows how to have fun.

And, seriously, I have Parkinson's disease to thank for all of this. I'm a lucky guy.

I finished in 4:30:32. It was the fastest of the six marathons I ran during these weeks. Shalane finished in 2:33:32 so I met the watered-down factor of two goal of mine in five of the six marathons that we both ran.

I met everyone back at the Airbnb, managing the four-story walkup without much trouble. Tom and Sue needed to head back to their home in Pennsylvania. Bob had left the city for his home in Westhampton after finishing his bicycle escort job. The rest of us went to Stout for the Team Fox postrace party. Team Fox had graciously extended the invitation to anyone associated with the runners so what was left of my entourage joined in.

Team Fox put on a sweet party, making me wistful for the ones that I missed in Chicago and Boston. Liz Diemer and her whole team were there and as runners entered the restaurant, they all cheered and clapped for them and a warm round of hugs were exchanged. Given that it was a lot of work to make marathon day special, I believe that they were happy and relieved that the day had come off so well for everyone.

I also caught up with Bill Bucklew again and met his wife, Heidi, who with this race finished her first marathon. She was happy and proud of her accomplishment but very clearly had decided that this was a "one-and-done" thing. No more marathon plans for her. Bill and I plan to keep in touch. He'll no doubt be keeping up his string of off-the-charts challenges and so perhaps I will join him on some in the future.

It was a long day and we still had some driving to do so, with another warm round of hugs, we were off.

After the postrace party my sister, Marcia, drove me, Charlotte, and Pat to her home in Stony Brook on the north shore of Long Island. Lynn and Kinsey stayed on in the city. Before Charlotte and Pat drove off to their homes out east, we celebrated again with a cake that had, surprise, a 'Joe Head' printed onto the frosting.

I spent the night with Marcia's family and then we drove together out to Greenport to see our mom. Along the way, Chris Hatler of *Runner's World* called and we conducted the interview by phone. Chris' very complimentary article was published on the *RW* digital feed the following day.[1]

Mom was happy to see us. She is already the celebrity at the facility what with 12 children, 27 grandchildren, and 15 great grandchildren and counting. Now she has bragging rights accorded to her by my feat, and for good measure Marcia and I affixed a yardstick-mounted 'Joe Head' to the back of her wheelchair. To me it looked kind of creepy but Mom loved it.

After our visit, Scott Hanson called from *The Seattle Times* and we conducted that interview by phone as well. I was rather pleased with Scott's article as it got four columns in the following Sunday's sports section replete with color photos.[2] I had the article mounted and sent it to Mom because that's what one does for Mom.

I had one other contact from the media after the race. Julie Sapper and Lisa Levin of *Run Farther & Faster* interviewed me for their podcast later in the month.[3] They specialize in helping runners prepare for the Boston Marathon, but they were inspired by my 2021 WMM challenge. I met up with them and some of their clients just before the 2022 Boston Marathon in April. Julie and Lisa introduced me as "the other guy who did what Shalane Flanagan did." Sweet.

After my visit with Mom, Marcia drove me to the train, which I took back into the city to get together with Lynn for dinner. On Tuesday morning, I took a last run in Central Park while my marathon medal was engraved with my name and finish time. Later that evening, Lynn and I flew back home to Seattle.

On Wednesday, three days after the race, I published the NYC Marathon recap to my blog. The adventure had come to its inevitable and satisfying conclusion.

And it really was over. Although Tokyo did admit some elite international runners to the March 6, 2022 race, it was virtually impossible for ordinary international runners to get into Japan. My sixth star would have to wait until 2023 at the earliest.

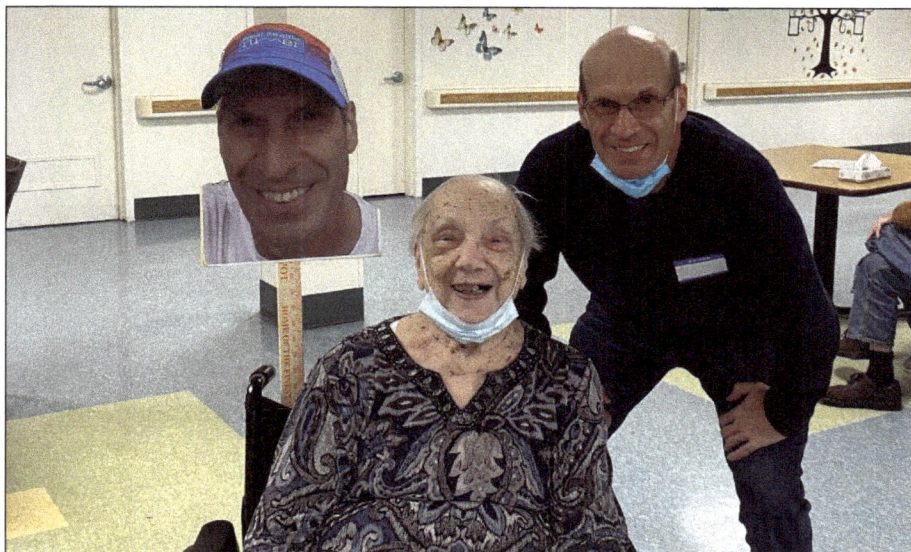

The day after the New York City Marathon I went to the San Simeon Center for Nursing and Rehabilitation in Greenport, Long Island to visit with my mother, Martha Drake. My sister, Marcia, and I brought along one of the 'Joe Heads' for Mom and we attached it to her wheelchair much to her delight (© M. Brandeau).

17

Run On Ahead

While in New York City, on the Friday before Sunday's marathon, Kinsey and I went to a presentation at MJFF headquarters led by Susanna Wach, an on-the-ground ambassador for the foundation. Kinsey has a degree in Biochemistry and is well-versed in the disciplines discussed. The presentation focused on recent developments and the pipeline of promising therapies for treating and potentially curing Parkinson's disease.

Alpha-synuclein, for example, is getting a lot of attention lately. Alpha-synuclein is a sticky protein that misfolds and aggregates in the brain of PD patients similar to the plaques found in Alzheimer's sufferers. One exciting line of research is the potential for a vaccine that inoculates against the accumulation of alpha-synuclein.[1,2]

It was gratifying to get some insight into how the money I've been raising through these marathons is contributing to a future world without Parkinson's disease. There is a substantial pipeline of potential solutions in process.

Yet, as promising as the pipeline may be, who knows how long it may take to develop a clinically usable cure? Years? Decades? What do newly diagnosed PD patients do until then?

I was particularly interested in progress toward a definitive clinical test for PD. I'd read of Joy Milne, the lady who can smell Parkinson's,* and was pleased to find out that a group at Harvard was working with her to develop a gas chromatograph-based artificial nose (GC-nose) that would sniff out the disease.[3,4] There's also been

---

*Joy Milne's story is fascinating. She has a powerful sense of smell that until recently she was not aware of. Ten years into her marriage with her husband, Les, she noticed that he began to smell different and over time Les displayed Parkinson's symptoms. When they went together to a PD support group it all started to make sense. Parkinson's has a smell, everyone in the support group had it to varying extents, and Joy alone could smell it. Given that Joy could smell PD well before symptoms manifested suggests that a powerful early clinical diagnostic for PD could be developed.

progress toward a biomarker to detect and track the progression of alpha-synuclein in live PD patients.[5,6]

My thinking is that until a cure has been identified, it's critical for those who have PD to begin therapies that are available today in order to slow its progression. The disease may progress 5 to 10 years unchecked before motor symptoms send the patient to a neurologist. Without an early definitive diagnosis, that's 5 to 10 years lost that could have been put to better use so that, when the cure comes, the patient would be in that much better shape to capitalize on it.

I recently caught up with Susanna Wach again and she reported that research toward early detection of PD is now a key focus of MJFF.

To the best of my knowledge and experience, for now, vigorous aerobic exercise is the only therapy we've got that has been proven to slow the disease progression. I would love to see more PD patients become motivated to start running before the disease becomes unbearable. As I've said before, it's been a game changer for me. But without a quantitative clinical test such a prospect is unlikely or nearly impossible.

I make no claims to be an expert in neurology. All I have is my personal experience with PD, a layman's understanding of the disease and how the brain deals with it, and a desire to learn more. I'll never claim that what works for me will work for all Parkies; I don't have the necessary credentials. Nonetheless, I think that it's a worthwhile place to start.

To recap, vigorous aerobic exercise has been proven to slow the progression of the disease. From what I've read in the professional literature, that's a view that has become generally accepted. I'm not sure if it stops the progression, though, so I make the best of it while I can.

More speculative is the proposition that exercise also stimulates the reward circuits of the brain and that this stimulation helps to overcome the mental challenge of putting in the long hours of exercise that may be needed to stall the progression. Works for me, though.

And here's another feature of my approach that I feel compelled to highlight because it may be useful to others in similar circumstances: It's been extremely valuable to me to set into motion an audacious goal and tell my loved ones about it.

This may have been the work of the invisible hand again. I don't know. It has a good track record. But for all I know, the invisible hand has really just been my brain all this time doing its job.

I couldn't do the 2021 WMM on my own. And I didn't need to. Because laying down a challenge of this magnitude energized a whole host of accomplices who embraced the life-affirming character of the journey. Friends, family, and new acquaintances I met along the way were inspired by my quest and shared in my successes, winced at my stumbles, contributed financially to my campaign, and just decided to be there with me. That's love and it's mighty.

I can't overstate how important this is to a PD patient. There's no quantifying it but I'm certain that my dopamine levels soared. All along the way I felt fantastic even when enduring some of the more painful stretches of the races. Sure, it's my brain that generated the additional dopamine, but it was the love from others that booted up the machine and sent it into overdrive.

As I write this, it's been months since returning from New York City and the elation has diminished somewhat. But I don't care. I know how to bring it all back again. I just need to pick another ridiculous quest and attack it with cheerful, stubborn resolve. I'm fairly certain that at least some of my 2021 WMM support team would come along for the ride. And very likely there'll be unexpected thrills and new friends along the way.

I'll have to ask when I run into them, but I suspect that Bill Bucklew, Jimmy Choi, Brett Parker, and others have already figured out the benefit of committing to over-the-top goals.

Although I expect to keep up the running, I have a feeling that running isn't the only activity that works here. For example, the simple act of putting these words to the page knowing that there are readers enjoying them is enormously satisfying. Certainly, I should consider branching out. Kinsey has already pointed out to me that running has become my new element at the expense of a broader sense of community. She would rather not see me remain so single-minded.

Notwithstanding, this challenge has earned me my 15 minutes of fame. My family and I have appeared live, in online digital media, and in print in the local newspaper. Heck, I should be able to milk this for a dopamine pick-me-up at gatherings of friends and family for decades, long after I'm no longer able to execute on audacious goals.

It'll be like what Don Larsen, an otherwise ordinary player who pitched the only perfect game in World Series history, said when asked if he ever tired of speaking about it: "No, why should I?"

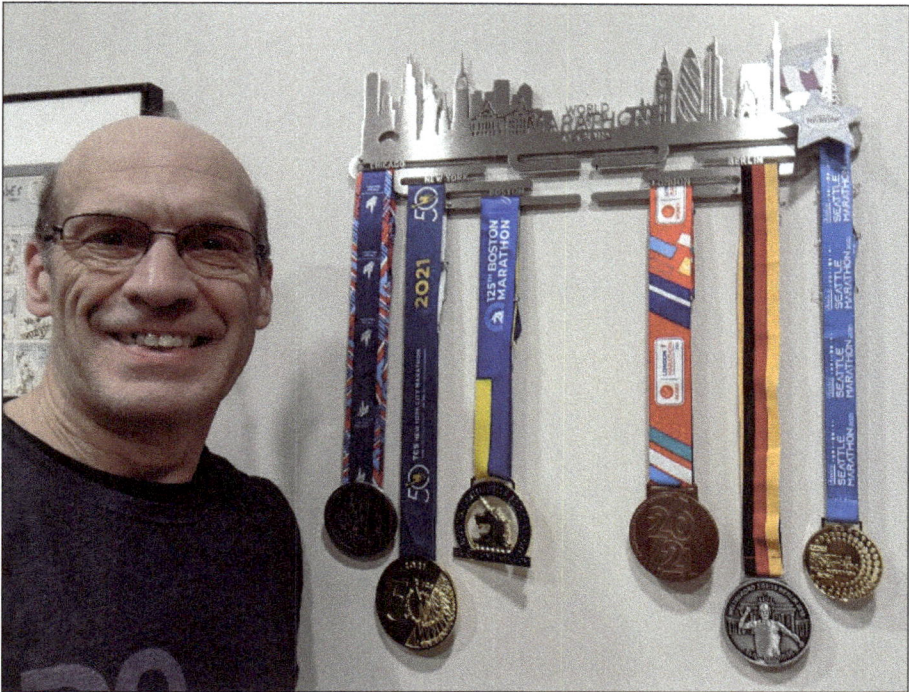

Posing with my medals from the 2021 WMM. The medal hanger was a gift from Lori and Tim McConnell of West Seattle Runner. Note the Seattle Marathon medal hanging to the far right in place of the Tokyo Marathon medal. Someday I will run in the Tokyo Marathon and its medal will replace the Seattle medal and in the center of the hanger will go the elusive Six Star Medal (© J. Drake).

Acknowledgements

As was the case with running the 2021 World Marathon Majors, I could not have written this book on my own. Many people provided the encouragement I needed, often with timing that was otherworldly. How did they know to push me along at the very moments when my motivation had flagged?

Howard Kolodny, Barb Kline-Schoder, and Ed Laufer reviewed an early draft of my first blog post. Their input convinced me that my writing style would not be an embarrassment. Tory Bers and Thelma Reese read through a first draft of my manuscript. I greatly appreciate their enthusiasm. Without it, I may not have put in the additional work required to transform that first effort into this book. Even then, as I became more aware of the enormity of the task required to publish and found my resolve fading, Grace-Lee Park appeared as if on cue and urged me on.

However, these folks are all longtime friends of mine and I have come to expect kindness from them. I sensed that I needed an independent review to point out where the manuscript needed work. The invisible hand directed me to a highly experienced editor, Liz Radojkovic. I tasked Liz with helping me make this book as good as it can be and urged her to be as ruthless as necessary. Being unkind is not in Liz's nature either, however. She graciously pointed out the manuscript's strengths and weaknesses and tactfully noted some of the less appealing quirks in my prose. Together we accomplished what we set out to do.

I thank Lori and Tim McConnell for ignoring my inexperience and hiring me to work at their wonderful shop, West Seattle Runner (WSR). Together with their store manager, Ferguson Mitchell, they opened my eyes to the world of running. Through WSR I met other local runners—Mike Marshino, Erika Whinihan, and Kelly Wright—who followed me on Strava and applauded my training efforts.

The Michael J. Fox Foundation (MJFF) provided me with entries to three of the marathons. Without MJFF's support it would not have been possible to race in all six of the marathons. In addition, the people I met at MJFF and Team Fox (Liz Berger, Colleen Bearsto, Katie Casamassina, Liz Diemer, Mary Havlock, Austyn Marks, Darryn Pulanco, and Susanna Wach) have been outstanding in their support for my effort. For a team that is working diligently to eliminate their jobs, they are the most dedicated, charming, and enthusiastic bunch that one could ever hope to meet.

In addition, I am thankful to the other Team Fox runners and their support people who shared with me their motivations for contributing to Parkinson's research: Michael Blum; Heidi and Bill Bucklew; Caroline Hershey and Natan Edelsburg; Inga, Rick, Julia, and Eric Jones; Eric Gesimondo; Melissa Loh; John McPhee; Jeremiah and Anne Marie Mushen; and Aaron Parker.

Crossing paths with other runners and their support people was an unexpected delight and I hope that we meet again. I list them here (alphabetically) and apologize to anyone I have missed: Dorothea Donelan Avery; Ed and Claire Bacher; Suzanne Barron; Sue Bilotta; Maureen Donelan; Jess Dorrington; Stephen Evans; Lisa Levin; Tess Newland; Rosie O'Sullivan; John Pasdois; Carol and John Porter; Brendan Reilly; Vitor Rodrigues; Karyn and Mark Ryan; Julie Sapper; Jan Sizer; Bryon Solberg; Carita Wegner; Brooke (Sizer), Cooper, and James Williamson.

Laura Paulus and Samantha Miller were instrumental in gaining me access to media outlets. Thank you for allowing me my 15 minutes of fame.

I appreciate the journalists who helped me to get the story of my approach of dealing with Parkinson's disease out to the world: Scott Hanson, Chris Hatler, Nick Kosir, and Marissa Torres. You have already helped many people suffering from this relentless disease by simply allowing me a forum for relating my strategy for it.

Sincerest thanks to the Drake family members (Pat, Bob, Marcia, Tom, Sue, Chris, Samantha, Charlotte, Lynn, and Kinsey) who made the trek to New York City to cheer me on and to proliferate 'Joe Heads' throughout Manhattan. Pat, an artist, also enthusiastically created this book's cover illustration for me. The collaboration was almost more enjoyable than the result of her work.

Dr. Benjamin Podemski did me the great favor of reading my manuscript and validating the medical science of Parkinson's disease described therein. It was a major milestone for me to obtain his approval and support.

I appreciate Martin Johannson at the Donders Institute for Brain, Cognition, and Behavior in the Netherlands for taking the time to answer my email queries about his work on the effect of exercise on Parkinson's patients.

Dozens of friends and neighbors followed me through my training plan, read my blog, contributed to my MJFF charitable campaign, and tracked me on race day. I am afraid that if I attempted to name all of you, I would miss someone. Suffice to say that I remember how wonderful you have been throughout this journey and I am forever grateful. However, I do wish to give heartfelt shoutouts to Louise and Steve Dunn-Massey for hosting me in England and to Darien Wood, Ela Barbaris, and their son, Max, for doing the same in Boston. Additionally, special thanks to Gail Foelsch and Ron Reade. Without fail, regardless of the city I was in, early morning of any given race day they would text or email me with well wishes for the day's upcoming marathon.

I owe thanks to the celebrities who unwittingly provided cameo roles to my story: Shalane Flanagan, Kyrsten Sinema, and Greta Thunberg. You've added a rich and surreal element to this already unpredictable tale.

Finally, I wish to thank my wife and my children for allowing me the opportunity to see this challenge through. Lynn, Aidan, and Kinsey, I love you to the moon and back.

Notes

Chapter 2. A Mystery

1. T. B. Stoker and J. C. Greenland, *Parkinson's disease*, 2018.
2. C. E. Clarke, Parkinson's disease, 2007.
3. Michael J. Fox Foundation, Parkinson's 101.
4. Z. Murphy, Parkinson's Disease | Clinical Presentation | Part 1, *YouTube*, 2017.
5. Z. Murphy, Parkinson's Disease | Causes and Pathophysiology | Part 2, *YouTube*, 2017.
6. Z. Murphy, Parkinson's Disease | Pharmacological Treatments | Part 3, *YouTube*, 2017.
7. Z. Murphy, Parkinson's disease, Part 3, 2017.
8. T. B. Stoker and J. C. Greenland, *Parkinson's disease*, 2018.
9. R. Dolhun, Ask the MD: Myths about levodopa, 2017.
10. W. Poewe, A. Antonini, J. C. Zijlmans, P. R. Burkhard, and F. Vingerhoets, Levodopa in the treatment of Parkinson's disease, 2010.
11. Michael J. Fox Foundation, Exercise.

Chapter 3. Learning to Run

1. Runners get a lot of practice with the metric system. The shorter organized road races are usually in metric distances, 5 and 10 kilometers, and usually abbreviated to 5K and 10K. A 5K race is 3.1 miles, 10K is 6.2 miles. Longer races like the marathon have historically used the Imperial system for measurement although depending on where they're held, they can be measurement schizophrenic. It's not uncommon for distance markers of both systems to be set up along the route (e.g., at every mile increment and at every 5K increment).
2. Finish time for marathons are usually given in either the "h:mm:ss.s" format or, briefly, "h:mm." Mile pace times, however, typically use the "mm:ss" time format. It's important to keep track of context to know what format is in play when discussing such things with a runner.
3. J. McGuire, How to run a marathon–Free marathon training plans for every kind of runner. *Runner's World*, 2022.
4. Runner's World, Runner's World training pace calculator, *Runner's World*, 2018.
5. A. Delacruz, Running form, *McMillan Running*.
6. A Google search on "posture cadence foot strike" yields some nice videos that demonstrate proper running form.
7. P. Dobos, The 180 steps per minute running myth, *EndurElite*.
8. A. Delacruz, Running form, *McMillan Running*.
9. C. Heffernan, The history of carbohydrate loading, *Physical Culture Study*, 2019.
10. A. Anderson, Fueling before, during & after a marathon, *Marine Corps Marathon*, 2020.
11. P. N. Bede, How to carb-load for marathon week, *Runner's World*, 2014.

12. Wikipedia Sourced, Gatorade.
13. D.J. Casa, Proper hydration for distance running–Identifying individual fluid needs, 2002.

Chapter 4. Escalating Goals

1. Abbott World Marathon Majors, https://www.worldmarathonmajors.com/
2. Abbott World Marathon Majors, Six Star finishers facts, 2022.
3. T. Gilliam and T. Jones (Directors). *Monty python and the holy grail*, 1975.
4. The purchase of carbon offsets is a way to decrease your personal carbon footprint. The dollars spent to buy the offsets fund programs that move the planet closer to carbon neutrality (i.e., reforestation, renewable energy projects, etc.). I purchased my offsets from TerraPass (www.terrapass.com) but there are others to choose from. TerraPass has a calculator on its website whereby estimated carbon usage is entered (i.e., planned airline flights, gas stoves, miles driven in gas powered cars, etc.) and it spits out the number of offsets required (and their cost) to neutralize those emissions. After buying them, TerraPass sent me a certificate that demonstrated my concern for the planet.
5. "How to Run the World Marathon Majors If You're Not an Elite," *The Runner Beans*, 2020.
6. The Expo is a fixture of most big city marathons. Its primary function is to orient participants to the event's protocol and to distribute race packets that include the runner's race bib, T-shirt, and swag. Expos usually include an exhibition hall as well where presentations are made and vendors hawk running-related equipment, apparel, and nutritional supplies.
7. Tokyo Marathon Race Director, Foreign runners excluded from Tokyo Marathon, 2021.

Chapter 5. Team Fox

1. Michael J. Fox, *Lucky man*, 2002.
2. Michael J. Fox Foundation, Home page, 2022.
3. Michael J. Fox Foundation, Strong pipeline of Parkinson's treatments, 2021.
4. Michael J. Fox, *No time like the future*, 2020.
5. Michael J. Fox Foundation, Be a fundraiser, 2022.
6. K. McCarrick, Walking 2,500 miles to close the gap on a cure, 2017.
7. B. Bucklew, Failure is the option, 2018.
8. Walk4Parkinsons, The long walk for Parkinson's, 2021.
9. A. Gardner, 7 marathons, 7 days, 7 continents and one man with Parkinson's, 2018.
10. Michael J. Fox Foundation, Jimmy Choi.
11. J. Choi, What I learned from "American Ninja Warrior" about living with Parkinson's, 2019.
12. J. Drake, Joe's gotta run (blog), 2021.

Chapter 6. A Customized Training Plan

1. Marathon Guide, *Boston Marathon qualifying races–Most likely to qualify*, 2019.
2. D. Robb, An improved GAP model, 2017. Strava uses runners' heartrate data to equate effort levels for a graded verses flat course (i.e., equivalent heartrate pace).
3. B. Hamilton, How to run downhill the right way, 2021.
4. J. Shaw, The secrets to downhill running fast, 2019.
5. W. Y. Sanchez, Sen. Kyrsten Sinema returns to Capitol Hill after breaking foot during marathon, 2021.
6. Spoiler Alert! Only about 24,000 runners applied for the 30,000 openings in the 2022 Boston Marathon. The smaller pool of applicants may have been due to continued COVID-19 concerns or maybe because the 2021 race was a mere six months earlier. In any event, for the first time since 2013 there was no cutoff time imposed; all valid BQ's were accepted. In addition, the qualifying window was extended backward to September 1, 2019. In other words, I was in but I could've done it without the Tunnel Marathon; my December 2019 CIM finish time alone qualified me.
7. F. Shaffer and J. P. Ginsberg, An overview of heart rate variability metrics and norms, 2017.

Chapter 7. Clues

1. Michael J. Fox Foundation, Parkinson's 101.
2. T. B. Stoker and J. C. Greenland, *Parkinson's disease*, 2018.
3. The animal model used to study Parkinson's disease is created by exposing mice to the neurotoxin MPTP. After exposure, the mice demonstrate Parkinson's-like symptoms.
4. M. Cone, Rural well water linked to Parkinson's disease, 2009.
5. K. E. Murros, V. A. Huynh, T. M. Takala, and P. E. Saris, Desulfovibrio bacteria are associated with Parkinson's disease, 2021.
6. Z. Murphy, Parkinson's disease, Part 3, 2017.
7. A. D. Wong, M. Ye, A. F. Levy, J. D. Rothstein, D. E. Bergles, and P. C. Searson, The blood-brain barrier, 2013.
8. Z. Murphy, Parkinson's disease, Part 3, 2017.
9. Z. Murphy, Parkinson's disease, Part 3, 2017.
10. D. Jiang, M. Li, L. Jiang, X. Chen, and X. Zhou, Comparison of selegiline and levodopa combination therapy versus levodopa monotherapy in the treatment of Parkinson's disease, 2019.
11. Y. Tan, P. Jenner, S. Chen, Monoamine Oxidase-B inhibitors for the treatment of Parkinson's disease, 2022.
12. S. Mantri, M. Lepore, B. Edison, M. Daeschler, C. Kopil, C. Marras, and L. Chahine, The experience of OFF periods in Parkinson's disease, 2021.
13. T. Carvalho, *Parkinson's News Today*, 2022.

14. Acorda Therapeutics, Inbrija, 2022.
15. D. Jiang, M. Li, L. Jiang, X. Chen, and X. Zhou, Comparison of selegiline and levodopa combination therapy, 2019.
16. A. Ni and C. Ernst, Evidence that substantia nigra pars compacta dopaminergic neurons are selectively vulnerable to oxidative stress because they are highly metabolically active, 2022.
17. H.-C. Cheng, C. M. Ulane, and R. E. Burke, Clinical progression in Parkinson's disease and the neurobiology of axons, 2010.
18. T. B. Stoker and J. C. Greenland, *Parkinson's disease*, 2018.
19. Parkinson's UK, Dystonia and muscle cramps, 2018.
20. Michael J. Fox Foundation, Parkinson's 101.
21. Michael J. Fox Foundation, Exercise.
22. N. Doidge, *The brain's way of healing*, 2016.
23. J. Pepper, *Reverse Parkinson's disease*, 2011.
24. N. Doidge, *The brain's way of healing*, 2016.
25. N. Doidge, *The brain's way of healing*, 2016.
26. M. Schenkman, C. Moore, W. Kohrt, D. Hall, A. Delitto, C. Comella, D. Josbeno, C. Christiansen, B. Berman, B. Kluger, E. Melanson, S. Jain, J. Robichaud, C. Poon, and D. Corcos, Effect of high-intensity treadmill exercise on motor symptoms in patients with De Novo Parkinson disease, 2018.
27. W. Suzuki, The brain-changing benefits of exercise, 2017.
28. M. Johansson, I. Cameron, N. Van der Kolk, N. de Vries, E. Klimars, I. Toni, B. Bloem, and R. Helmich, Aerobic exercise alters brain function and structure in Parkinson's disease, 2022.
29. F. P. Manfredsson, N. P. Polinski, T. Subramanian, N. Boulis, D. R. Wakeman, and R. J. Mandel, The future of GDNF in Parkinson's disease, 2020.
30. F. P. Manfredsson, N. P. Polinski, T. Subramanian, N. Boulis, D. R. Wakeman, and R. J. Mandel, The future of GDNF, 2020.
31. M. Johansson, I. Cameron, N. Van der Kolk, N. de Vries, E. Klimars, I. Toni, B. Bloem, and R. Helmich, Aerobic exercise, 2022.
32. M. Schenkman, C. Moore, W. Kohrt, D. Hall, A. Delitto, C. Comella, D. Josbeno, C. Christiansen, B. Berman, B. Kluger, E. Melanson, S. Jain, J. Robichaud, C. Poon, and D. Corcos, Effect of high-intensity treadmill exercise, 2018.
33. M. Johansson, I. Cameron, N. Van der Kolk, N. de Vries, E. Klimars, I. Toni, B. Bloem, and R. Helmich, Aerobic exercise, 2022.

Chapter 8. The Killer App

1. Runner's World, This is why Kipchoge smiles when he runs (and why you should be doing it too), 2018.
2. Wikipedia Sourced, Hysterical strength.
3. W. Suzuki, The brain-changing benefits of exercise, 2017.

Chapter 9. The Pandemic Gauntlet

1. Tokyo Marathon Race Director, Foreign runners excluded from Tokyo Marathon, 2021.
2. C. Hatler, The 2021 Tokyo Marathon has been postponed from October to March, 2021.
3. S. R. Kelleher, It's official: EU recommends travel ban for American tourists, 2021.

Chapter 10. The Inscrutable Media

1. T. Dutch, Retired elite runner Shalane Flanagan announces her goal to run 6 World Marathons in 42 Days, each in under 3 hours, 2021.
2. L. Miller, Running legend Shalane Flanagan will take on all 6 Major Marathons this fall, 2021.
3. NBC, Shalane Flanagan to run six marathons in 42 days, including Bank of America Chicago Marathon, 2021.

Chapter 11. Berlin

1. Suzanne appeared to bond with me because of my name. She's worked in the movie industry and knew of another Joe Drake who was known to be a good guy. That Joe Drake produced the films *Juno*, *Harold and Kumar Go to White Castle*, and *This is the End* and many others.
2. GreenwichFreePress, At 67, Greenwich running club's Rose O'Sullivan shares the journey of her 100 marathons, 2018.
3. K. Laub and F. Jordans, Greta Thunberg joins climate rally in Germany ahead of election, 2021.

Chapter 12. London

1. C. Giuliani and A. Peri, Effects of hyponatremia on the brain, 2014.
2. Mayo Clinic, Hyponatremia.
3. C. Almond, A. Shin, E. Fortescue, R. Mannix, D. Wypij, B. Binstadt, C. Duncan, D. Olson, A. Salerno, J. Newburger, and D. Greenes, Hyponatremia among runners in the Boston Marathon, 2005.
4. W. Zevon, Werewolves of London, 1978.
5. Max Shinsheimer is a literary agent and although I didn't find out his connection to PD, he did help me later on with some guidance on positioning this book to be published.

Chapter 13. The Doubleheader: Chicago–Boston

1. Foundation for Sarcoidosis Research, What is sarcoidosis?
2. B. Navi, Prior stroke and other cerebrovascular risk factors linked with Parkinson's disease, 2019.
3. It's that measurement schizophrenia thing again. Despite the official marathon distance being in miles, a runner's progress is tracked with timing mats placed at 5-kilometer intervals. When a runner steps on the mat a signal is sent to the tracking app thus alerting the runner's supporters of their status. Something must have gone wrong with the signal from the 40-kilometer timing mat.

Chapter 14. Tokyo aka Seattle

1. A. Reese, READER REPORT: Joe's 'virtual Tokyo' in West Seattle, 2021.

Chapter 15. Team 50

1. Press Releases, Team 50 to represent stories of most inspiring runners at 50th running of the TCS New York City Marathon on Sunday, November 7, 2021.

Chapter 16. New York City

1. C. Hatler, After being diagnosed with Parkinson's, he decided to run the World Marathon Majors, 2021.
2. S. Hanson, Joe Drake fights back against Parkinson's disease by running marathon after marathon, 2021.
3. L. Levin and J. Sapper, Episode 111: Shalane Flanagan was not the only one to complete six Marathon Majors in seven weeks . . . Meet Joe Drake, 2021.

Chapter 17. Run On Ahead

1. D. Jimenez, Parkinson's disease: Could a vaccine be on the horizon?, 2021.
2. M. Kuhl, Major deal pushes Parkinson's vaccine further in testing, 2021.
3. R. Gilbert, The smell of Parkinson's disease, 2019.
4. A. Spiegel and E. Renken, Her incredible sense of smell is helping scientists find new ways to diagnose disease, 2020.
5. D. Trevedi, E. Sinclair, Y. Xu, D. Sarkar, C. Walton-Doyle, C. Liscio, P. Banks, J. Milne, M. Silverdale, T. Kunath, R. Goodacre, and P. Barran, Discovery of volatile biomarkers of Parkinson's disease from Sebum, 2019.
6. K. Magana, News in context: Tool to visualize key Parkinson's protein in the brain enters human testing, 2021.

Bibliography

Abbott World Marathon Majors. (2022). Six Star finishers facts. Abbott World
    Marathon Majors.

Abbott World Marathon Majors. (n.d.). Retrieved from World Marathon
    Majors: https://www.worldmarathonmajors.com/

Acorda Therapeutics. (2022). Inbrija. Retrieved from https://www.inbrija.com/

Almond, C., Shin, A., Fortescue, E., Mannix, R., Wypij, D., Binstadt, B.,
    Duncan, C., Olson, D., Salerno, A., Newburger, J., & Greenes, D. (2005).
    Hyponatremia among runners in the Boston Marathon. *The New England
    Journal of Medicine*, (352), 1550–1556.

Anderson, A. (2020, March 5). Fueling before, during & after a marathon.
    Retrieved from *Marine Corps Marathon*: https://www.marinemarathon.
    com/blog/fueling-your-body#:~:text=A%20good%20rule%20of%20
    thumb,increase%20up%20to%200.75%20oz

Bede, P. N. (2014, April 16). How to carb-load for marathon week. Retrieved
    from *Runner's World*: https://www.runnersworld.com/nutrition-weight-
    loss/a20822836/how-to-carb-load-for-marathon-week/

Bucklew, B. (2018, June). Failure is the option. Retrieved from *TED*:
    https://www.ted.com/talks/bill_bucklew_failure_is_the_option

Carvalho, T. (2022, February 9). *Parkinson's News Today*. Retrieved from
    https://parkinsonsnewstoday.com/kynmobi-apomorphine-for-the-
    reduction-of-off-episodes-in-parkinsons

Casa, D. J. (2002). Proper hydration for distance running–Identifying
    individual fluid needs. University of Connecticut, Athletic Training
    Education. USA Track and Field.

Cheng, H.-C., Ulane, C. M., & Burke, R. E. (2010). Clinical progression in Parkinson's
    disease and the neurobiology of axons. *Annals of Neurology*, 1–19.

Choi, J. (2019, July 9). What I learned from "American Ninja Warrior" about
    living with Parkinson's disease. Retrieved from *The Michael J. Fox*

Foundation: https://www.michaeljfox.org/news/what-i-learned-american-ninja-warrior-about-living-parkinsons-disease

Clarke, C. E. (2007, September 1). Parkinson's disease. *Clinical Review*, 335, 441–445.

Cone, M. (2009, August 5). Rural well water linked to Parkinson's disease. Retrieved April 5, 2022, from *Scientific American*: https://www.scientificamerican.com/article/rural-well-water-insecticides-parkinsons-disease-california/

Delacruz, A. (n.d.). Running form. Retrieved from *McMillan Running*: https://www.mcmillanrunning.com/topic/running-form/

Dobos, P. (n.d.). The 180 steps per minute running myth. Retrieved from *EndurElite*: https://endurelite.com/blogs/free-nutrition-supplement-and-training-articles-for-runners-and-cyclists/the-180-steps-per-minute-running-myth

Doidge, N. (2016). *The brain's way of healing*. New York City: Penguin Books.

Dolhun, R. (2017, August 30). Ask the MD: Myths about levodopa. Retrieved from *The Michael J. Fox Foundation*: https://www.michaeljfox.org/news/ask-md-myths-about-levodopa

Drake, J. (2021). Joe's gotta run (blog). Retrieved from *Medium*: https://joesgottarun.medium.com/

Dutch, T. (2021, September 20). Retired elite runner Shalane Flanagan announces her goal to run 6 world marathons in 42 days, each in under 3 hours. Retrieved from *Self*: https://www.self.com/story/shalane-flanagan-2021-world-majors?fbclid=IwAR1PHiCuY3TAlUNJ3gFSLHl5GZf2FEh zjYO8282YzSHu0MkcHOBbQGgvFx8

Fox, M. J. (2002). *Lucky man: A memoir*. Hyperion.

Fox, M. J. (2008). *Always looking up: The adventures of an incurable optimist*. Hyperion.

Fox, M. J. (2010). *A funny thing happened on the way to the future: Twists and turns and lessons learned*. Hachette Books.

Fox, M. J. (2020). *No time like the future: An optimist considers mortality*. Flatiron Books.

Foundation for Sarcoidosis Research. (n.d.). What is sarcoidosis? Retrieved from *Foundation for Sarcoidosis Research*: https://www.stopsarcoidosis. org/what-is-sarcoidosis/

Gardner, A. (2018, February 11). 7 marathons, 7 days, 7 continents and one man with Parkinson's. Can he make it? Retrieved from *The Washington Post*: https://www.washingtonpost.com/national/health-science/7-marathons-7-days-7-continents-and-one-man-with-parkinsons-can-he-make-it/2018/02/09/ef39ce80-0c14-11e8-8b0d-891602206fb7_story.html

Gilbert, R. (2019, December 11). The smell of Parkinson's disease. Retrieved from *American Parkinson Disease Association*: https://www.apdaparkinson.org/article/the-smell-of-parkinsons-disease/

Gilliam, T., & Jones, T. (Directors). (1975, March 14). *Monty python and the holy grail* [Motion Picture].

Giuliani, C., & Peri, A. (2014, October 28). Effects of hyponatremia on the brain. *Journal of Clinical Medicine*, 3, 1163–1177. doi:10.3390/jcm3041163

GreenwichFreePress. (2018, April 9). At 67, Greenwich running club's Rose O'Sullivan shares the journey of her 100 marathons. Retrieved April 5, 2022, from *Greenwich Free Press*: https://greenwichfreepress.com/schools/at-67-greenwich-running-clubs-rose-osullivan-shares-the-journey-of-her-100-marathons-104527/

Hamilton, B. (2021, January 20). How to run downhill the right way. Retrieved from *Canadian Running*: https://runningmagazine.ca/sections/training/how-to-run-downhill-the-right-way/

Hanson, S. (2021, November 13). Joe Drake fights back against Parkinson's disease by running marathon after marathon. Retrieved from *The Seattle Times*: https://www.seattletimes.com/sports/other-sports/joe-drake-fights-back-against-parkinsons-disease-by-running-marathon-after-marathon/#comments

Hatler, C. (2021, November 9). After being diagnosed with Parkinson's, he decided to run the World Marathon Majors. Retrieved from *Runner's World*: https://www.runnersworld.com/runners-stories/a38200065/joe-drake-six-marathon-majors-parkinsons-disease/

Hatler, C. (2021, September 17). The 2021 Tokyo Marathon has been postponed from October to March. Retrieved April 5, 2022, from *Runner's World*: https://www.runnersworld.com/news/a37634144/2021-tokyo-marathon-postponed/

Heffernan, C. (2019, March 27). The history of carbohydrate loading. Retrieved from *Physical Culture Study*: https://physicalculturestudy.com/2019/03/27/the-history-of-carbohydrate-loading/

"How to Run the World Marathon Majors If You're Not an Elite." (2020, September 28). Retrieved from *The Runner Beans*: https://therunnerbeans.com/run-world-marathon-majors-when-non-elite/

Jiang, D., Li, M., Jiang, L., Chen, X., & Zhou, X. (2019). Comparison of selegiline and levodopa combination therapy versus levodopa monotherapy in the treatment of Parkinson's disease: A meta-analysis. *Aging Clin Exp Res.*, 769–779.

Jimenez, D. (2021, August 3). Parkinson's disease: Could a vaccine be on the horizon? Retrieved from *Pharmaceutical Technology*: https://www.pharmaceutical-technology.com/features/parkinsons-vaccine-disease/

Johansson, M., Cameron, I., Van der Kolk, N., de Vries, N., Klimars, E., Toni, I., Bloem, B., & Helmich, R. (2022). Aerobic exercise alters brain function and structure in Parkinson's disease: A randomized controlled trial. *Annals of Neurology*, 1–14.

Kelleher, S. R. (2021, August 31). It's official: E.U. recommends travel ban for American tourists. Retrieved from *Forbes*: https://www.forbes.com/sites/suzannerowankelleher/2021/08/30/its-official-eu-recommends-travel-ban-for-american-tourists/?sh=4eea512f3070

Kuhl, M. (2021, August 4). Major deal pushes Parkinson's vaccine further in testing. Retrieved from *The Michael J. Fox Foundation*: https://www.michaeljfox.org/news/major-deal-pushes-parkinsons-vaccine-further-testing

Langley, J., Huddleston, D., & Hu, X. (2020). Chapter 20–Detecting parkinsonian degeneration in lateroventral tier of substantia nigra pars compacta with MRI. In C. Martin, *Genetics, Neurology, Behavior, and Diet in Parkinson's Disease* (pp. 313–325). Academic Press.

Laub, K., & Jordans, F. (2021, September 24). Greta Thunberg joins climate rally in Germany ahead of election. Retrieved from *CTV News*: https://www.ctvnews.ca/climate-and-environment/greta-thunberg-joins-climate-rally-in-germany-ahead-of-election-1.5598768

Levin, L., & Sapper, J. (2021, November 19). Episode 111: Shalane Flanagan was not the only one to complete six Marathon Majors in seven weeks . . . Meet Joe Drake. Retrieved from *Run Farther & Faster–The Podcast with Coaches Lisa Levin and Julie Sapper*: https://podcasts.apple.com/us/podcast/episode-111-shalane-flanagan-was-not-the-only-one-to/id1438350876?i=1000542494796

Magana, K. (2021, February 26). News in context: Tool to visualize key Parkinson's protein in the brain enters human testing. Retrieved from *The Michael J. Fox Foundation*: https://www.michaeljfox.org/news/news-context-tool-visualize-key-parkinsons-protein-brain-enters-human-testing

Manfredsson, F. P., Polinski, N. P., Subramanian, T., Boulis, N., Wakeman, D. R., & Mandel, R. J. (2020, December). The future of GDNF in Parkinson's disease. *Frontiers in Aging Neuroscience, 12,* 1–6.

Mantri, S., Lepore, M., Edison, B., Daeschler, M., Kopil, C., Marras, C., and Chahine, L. (2021, July 19). The experience of OFF periods in Parkinson's disease: Descriptions, triggers, and alleviating factors. *J Patient Cent Res Rev., 8,* 232–238. doi: 10.17294/2330-0698.1836

Marathon Guide. (2019). Boston Marathon qualifying races–Most likely to qualify–2019. Retrieved from *Marathon Guide*: http://www.marathonguide.com/races/bostonmarathonqualifyingraces.cfm?Year=2019

Mayo Clinic. (n.d.). Hyponatremia. Retrieved from *Mayo Clinic*: https://www.mayoclinic.org/diseases-conditions/hyponatremia/symptoms-causes/syc-20373711

McCarrick, K. (2017, November 27). Walking 2,500 miles to close the gap on a cure. Retrieved from *The Michael J. Fox Foundation*: https://www.michaeljfox.org/news/walking-2500-miles-close-gap-cure

McGuire, J. (2022, January 19). How to run a marathon–Free marathon training plans for every kind of runner. Retrieved from *Runner's World*:

https://www.runnersworld.com/uk/training/marathon/a776459/
marathon-training-plans/

Michael J. Fox Foundation. (2021, April). Strong pipeline of Parkinson's
treatments. Retrieved from *The Michael J. Fox Foundation*:
https://www.michaeljfox.org/: https://www.michaeljfox.org/sites/
default/files/media/document/MJFF_Spring_2021_Pipeline_.pdf

Michael J. Fox Foundation. (2022). Be a fundraiser. Retrieved from *The Michael
J. Fox Foundation*: https://www.michaeljfox.org/be-fundraiser-0

Michael J. Fox Foundation. (2022, May 25). Exercise. Retrieved from *The
Michael J. Fox Foundation*: https://www.michaeljfox.org/news/exercise

Michael J. Fox Foundation. (2022, May 25). Home page. Retrieved from *The
Michael J. Fox Foundation*: https://www.michaeljfox.org/

Michael J. Fox Foundation. (n.d.). Jimmy Choi. Retrieved from *The Michael J.
Fox Foundation*: https://www.michaeljfox.org/bio/jimmy-choi

Michael J. Fox Foundation. (n.d.). Parkinson's 101. Retrieved from *The Michael
J. Fox Foundation*: https://www.michaeljfox.org/parkinsons-101

Miller, L. (2021, September 20). Running legend Shalane Flanagan will take
on all 6 Major Marathons this fall. Retrieved from *PopSugar*:
https://www.popsugar.com/fitness/shalane-flanagan-to-run-all-6-major-
marathons-in-fall-2021-48510957

Murphy, Z. (2017, March 31). Parkinson's Disease | Causes and
Pathophysiology | Part 2. Retrieved from *YouTube*:
https://www.youtube.com/watch?v=rFoc4ACFehQ

Murphy, Z. (2017, March 31). Parkinson's Disease | Clinical Presentation |
Part 1. Retrieved from *YouTube*: https://www.youtube.com/
watch?v=KWVJBg6SCoY

Murphy, Z. (2017, March 31). Parkinson's Disease | Pharmacological
Treatments | Part 3. Retrieved from *YouTube*: https://www.youtube.com/
watch?v=LJVcrvrFYJs

Murros, K. E., Huynh, V. A., Takala, T. M., & Saris, P. E. (2021, May 3).
Desulfovibrio bacteria are associated with Parkinson's disease.
Frontiers in Cellular and Infection Microbiology, 11, 1–10. doi:10.3389/
fcimb.2021.652617

National Library of Medicine. (2022, January 15). *NIH: National Library of Medicine: Selegiline*. Retrieved from *MedLine Plus*: https://medlineplus.gov/druginfo/meds/a697046.html

Navi, B. (2019, August 29). Prior stroke and other cerebrovascular risk factors linked with Parkinson's disease. Retrieved from *Weill Cornell Medicine*: https://news.weill.cornell.edu/news/2019/08/prior-stroke-and-other-cerebrovascular-risk-factors-linked-with-parkinson%E2%80%99s-disease

NBC. (2021, September 20). Shalane Flanagan to run six marathons in 42 days, including Bank of America Chicago Marathon. Retrieved from *NBC Chicago*: https://www.nbcchicago.com/news/sports/chicago-marathon/shalane-flanagan-to-run-six-marathons-in-42-days-including-bank-of-america-chicago-marathon/2617776/

Ni, A., & Ernst, C. (2022, March 4). Evidence that substantia nigra pars compacta dopaminergic neurons are selectively vulnerable to oxidative stress because they are highly metabolically active. *Frontiers in Cellular Neuroscience*, 1–8.

Parkinson's Foundation. (n.d.). Neuroprotective benefits of exercise. Retrieved from *Parkinson's Foundation*: https://www.parkinson.org/Understanding-Parkinsons/Treatment/Exercise/Neuroprotective-Benefits-of-Exercise

Parkinson's UK. (2018). Dystonia and muscle cramps. Retrieved from *Dystonia and muscle cramps*: https://www.parkinsons.org.uk/information-and-support/dystonia-and-muscle-cramps

Pepper, J. (2011). *Reverse Parkinson's disease*. Dorrance Publishing.

Poewe, W., Antonini, A., Zijlmans, J. C., Burkhard, P. R., & Vingerhoets, F. (2010, August 24). Levodopa in the treatment of Parkinson's disease: An old drug still going strong. *Clinical Interventions in Aging*, 229–238.

Press Releases. (2021, October 21). Team 50 to represent stories of most inspiring runners at 50th running of the TCS New York City Marathon on Sunday, November 7. Retrieved from *New York Road Runners | Media Center*: https://www.nyrr.org/media-center/press-release/20211021_team50

Reese, A. (2021, October 17). READER REPORT: Joe's 'virtual Tokyo' in West Seattle. Retrieved from *West Seattle Blog*: https://westseattleblog.com/2021/10/reader-report-joes-virtual-tokyo-in-west-seattle/

Robb, D. (2017, October 3). An improved GAP model. Retrieved from *Strava Engineering on Medium*: https://medium.com/strava-engineering/an-improved-gap-model-8b07ae8886c3

Runner's World. (2018, May 1). Runner's World's training pace calculator. Retrieved from *Runner's World*: https://www.runnersworld.com/uk/training/a761676/rws-training-pace-calculator/

Runner's World. (2018, November 2). This is why Kipchoge smiles when he runs (and why you should be doing it too). Retrieved from *Runner's World*: https://www.runnersworld.com/uk/training/motivation/a776539/how-smiling-improves-your-running/

Sanchez, W. Y. (2021, June 14). Sen. Kyrsten Sinema returns to Capitol Hill after breaking foot during marathon. Retrieved from *AZ Central*: https://www.azcentral.com/story/news/politics/arizona/2021/06/14/sen-kyrsten-sinema-breaks-foot-running-tunnel-marathon/7686682002/

Savica, R., Rocca, W., & Ahlskog, J. E. (2010). When does Parkinson disease start? *JAMA Neurology, 67*(7), 798–801.

Schenkman, M., Moore, C., Kohrt, W., Hall, D., Delitto, A., Comella, C., Josbeno, D., Christiansen, C., Berman, B., Kluger, B., Melanson, E., Jain, S., Robichaud, J., Poon, C., & Corcos, D. (2018, February). Effect of high-intensity treadmill exercise on motor symptoms in patients with De Novo Parkinson disease. *JAMA Neurology, 75*(2), 219–226.

Shaffer, F., & Ginsberg, J. P. (2017). An overview of heart rate variability metrics and norms. *Frontiers in Public Health, 5*(258), 1–17.

Shaw, J. (2019, June 10). The secrets to downhill running fast. Retrieved from *Triathlete*: https://www.triathlete.com/training/the-secrets-to-running-downhill-fast/

Spiegel, A., & Renken, E. (2020). Her incredible sense of smell is helping scientists find new ways to diagnose disease. Retrieved from *National Public Radio*: https://www.npr.org/sections/health-shots/2020/03/23/820274501/her-incredible-sense-of-smell-is-helping-scientists-find-new-ways-to-diagnose-disease

Stoker, T. B., & Greenland, J. C. (Eds.). (2018). *Parkinson's disease: Pathogenesis and clinical aspects.* Brisbane, Australia: Codon Publications.

Suzuki, W. (2017, October). The brain-changing benefits of exercise. Retrieved from *TED Ideas Worth Spreading*: https://www.ted.com/talks/wendy_suzuki_the_brain_changing_benefits_of_exercise

Tan, Y., Jenner, P., & Chen, S. (2022). Monoamine Oxidase-B inhibitors for the treatment of Parkinson's disease: Past, present, and future. *Journal of Parkinson's Disease*, 477–493.

Tokyo Marathon Race Director. (2021, June 17). Foreign runners excluded from Tokyo Marathon. Retrieved April 5, 2022, from *Association of International Marathons and Distance Races*: https://aims-worldrunning.org/articles/1767-foreign-runners-excluded-from-tokyo-marathon.html

Trevedi, D., Sinclair, E., Xu, Y., Sarkar, D., Walton-Doyle, C., Liscio, C., Banks, P., Milne, J., Silverdale, M., Kunath, T., Goodacre, R., & Barran, P. (2019, April 24). Discovery of volatile biomarkers of Parkinson's disease from Sebum. *ACS Central Science, 5*(4), 599–606.

Walk4Parkinsons. (2021). The long walk for Parkinson's. Retrieved from *Walk 4 Parkinson's*: https://walk4parkinsons.org/

Wikipedia Sourced. (n.d.). Hysterical strength. Retrieved from *Wikipedia*: https://en.wikipedia.org/wiki/Hysterical_strength

Wikipedia Sourced. (n.d.). Gatorade. Retrieved from *Wikipedia*: https://en.wikipedia.org/wiki/Gatorade

Wong, D. A., Ye, M., Levy, A. F., Rothstein, J. D., Bergles D. E., & Searson, P. C. (2013). The blood-brain barrier: An engineering perspective. *Frontiers in Neuroengineering.*

Zevon, W. (1978). Werewolves of London [Recorded by W. Zevon].